Welcome

If you've picked up this book it's likely that you're experiencing the early stages of perimenopause and want to know what's on the way. Either that or you're in the middle of 'the change' and are looking for advice about ways to ease some of your symptoms. Perhaps you want to support a friend or partner going through menopause and you want to understand more about it. Either way, there's something here for you.

From learning about the stages of menopause, how it's diagnosed and treated to managing symptoms and learning not just to cope but to thrive physically, mentally and socially, this book shows menopause is more than just hot flushes. Every woman's experience of menopause is unique, but a problem shared is a problem halved. Through sharing stories and information we can help each other. This book seeks to empower women to take control of their lives, to embrace the changes and find freedom through a new positive outlook.

LIVING WITH
Menopause

Future PLC Quay House, The Ambury, Bath, BA1 1UA

Bookazine Editorial
Editor **Zara Gaspar**
Senior Designer **Harriet Knight**
Senior Art Editor **Andy Downes**
Head of Art & Design **Greg Whitaker**
Editorial Director **Jon White**

Contributors
Lora Barnes, Sophie Barton, Rebecca Bradbury, Elizabeth Carr-Ellis, Ella Carter, Kate Codrington, Jo Cole, Natalie Denton, Jane Druker, Briony Duguid, Jenna Farmer, Jamie Frier, Bee Ginger, Janey Lee Grace, Lynnette Hecker, Adam Markiewicz, Joan McFadden, Dan Peel, Fiona Russell, Suzy Stanton

Cover images
Getty Images

Photography
Getty Images
All copyrights and trademarks are recognised and respected

Advertising
Media packs are available on request
Commercial Director **Clare Dove**

International
Head of Print Licensing **Rachel Shaw**
licensing@futurenet.com
www.futurecontenthub.com

Circulation
Head of Newstrade **Tim Mathers**

Production
Head of Production **Mark Constance**
Production Project Manager **Matthew Eglinton**
Advertising Production Manager **Joanne Crosby**
Digital Editions Controller **Jason Hudson**
Production Managers **Keely Miller, Nola Cokely, Vivienne Calvert, Fran Twentyman**

Printed in the UK

Distributed by Marketforce, 5 Churchill Place, Canary Wharf, London, E14 5HU
www.marketforce.co.uk Tel: 0203 787 9001

Living with Menopause First Edition (4882)
© 2022 Future Publishing Limited

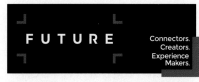

Future plc is a public company quoted on the London Stock Exchange (symbol: FUTR)
www.futureplc.com

Chief executive **Zillah Byng-Thorne**
Non-executive chairman **Richard Huntingford**
Chief financial officer **Penny Ladkin-Brand**

Tel +44 (0)1225 442 244

Widely Recycled

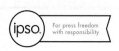

Contents

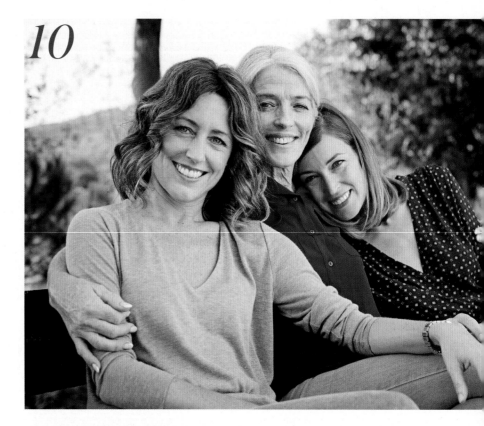

10

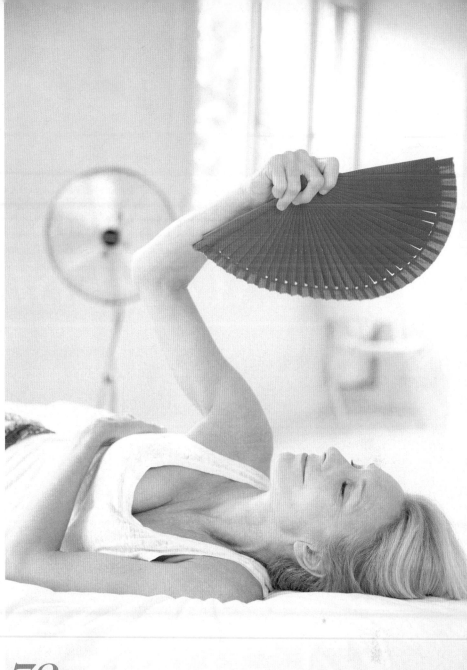

72

113

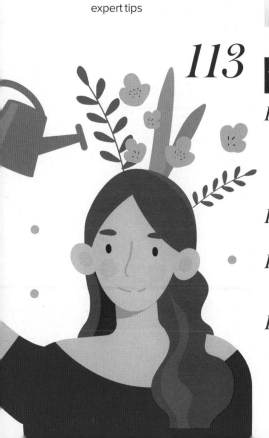

Introduction to
MENOPAUSE

Menopause doesn't have to be the end of a woman's best years – it can be the beginning

For many women, the **menopause can be a concerning time.** Whether it's worries about their physical health, mental health or relationships, there are just so many unknowns that hit at the same time as those hot flushes. There are myriad myths about the change, some of which are true, some of which are false and some of which are grossly exaggerated.

All of these can turn a perfectly natural time in a woman's life into something unnecessarily scary. There are many who say it shouldn't be called meno-pause, but meno-start, as it represents the next, exciting stage in a woman's life. Although there are obvious difficulties, this book will demonstrate why menopause is something that should be embraced rather than feared.

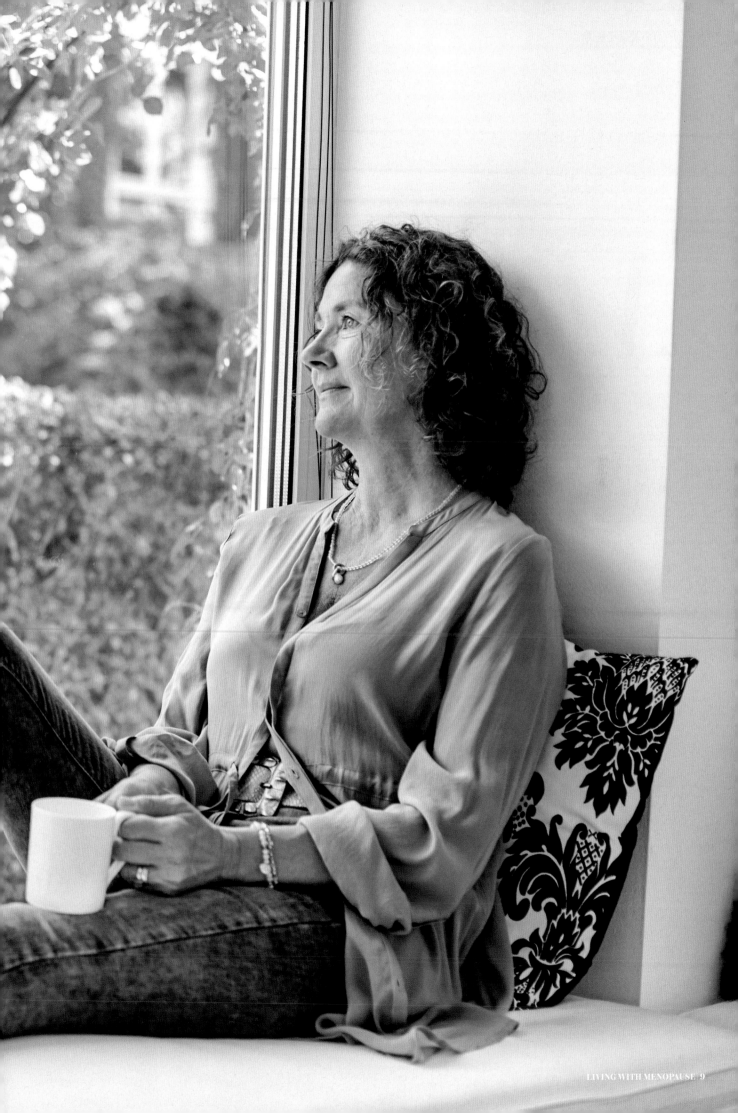

WHAT IS THE
Menopause?

One of life's biggest transitions is rarely spoken about, but
the menopause doesn't have to remain a mystery

Words by Rebecca Bradbury

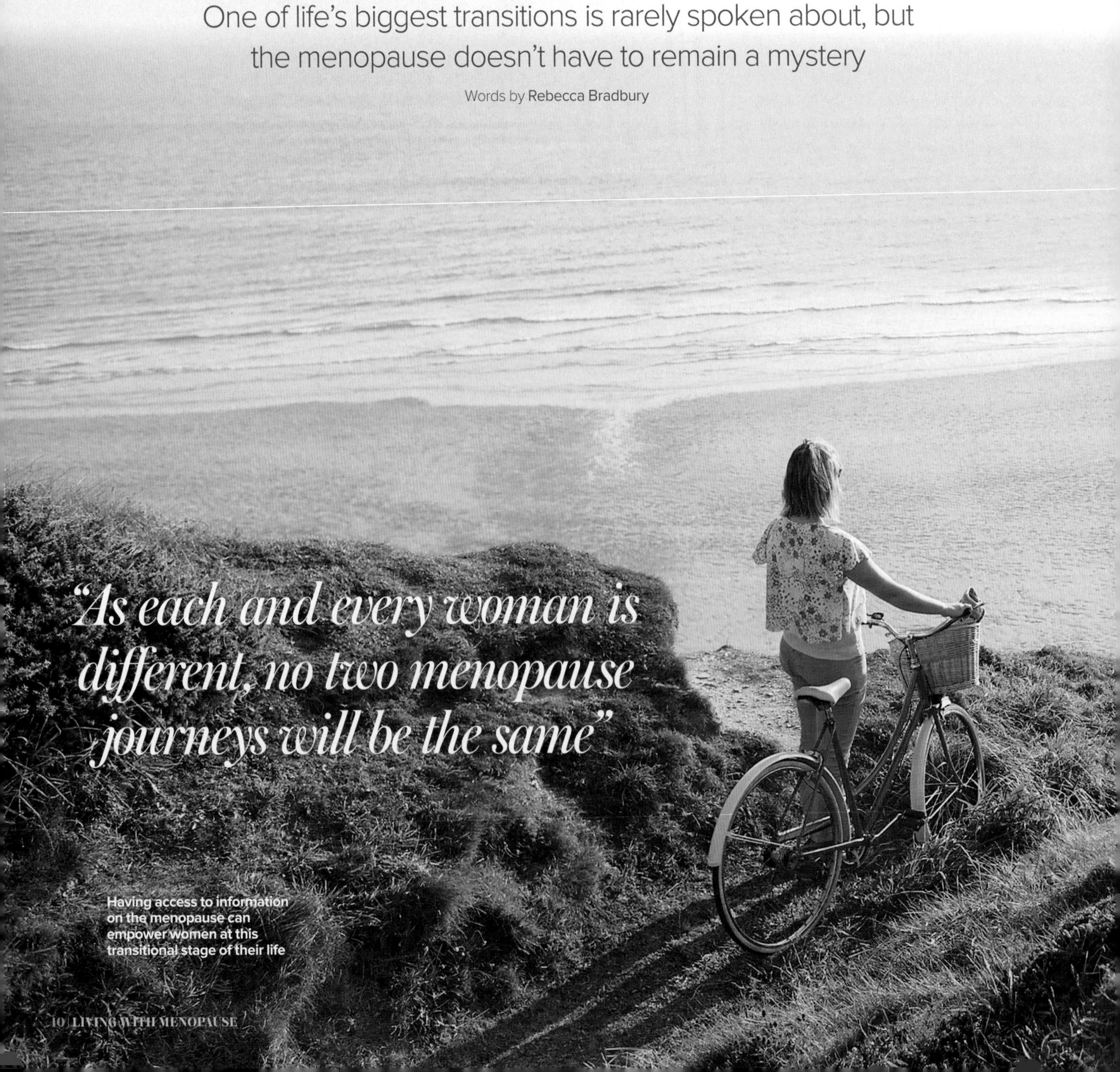

*"As each and every woman is
different, no two menopause
journeys will be the same"*

Having access to information
on the menopause can
empower women at this
transitional stage of their life

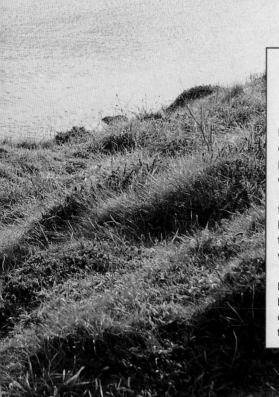

Menopause is one of those events every woman knows will eventually come, but doesn't want to think much about. Yet learning how it could affect both body and mind can help banish fears surrounding the transition and make the process far less stressful.

But what exactly is going on? As women approach their late 30s, their ovaries start making less oestrogen and progesterone – the hormones that regulate menstruation – and fertility declines. Periods will become increasingly irregular and eventually stop completely. The point at which a woman has not had a period for 12 consecutive months is called the menopause, and usually occurs between the ages of 45 and 55.

Note how the menopause is a point in time. It's often mistaken as the period of time leading up to this moment. However, this stage is called the perimenopause.

For a minority of women, hormones aren't to blame, as the menopause can be triggered by chemotherapy or radiotherapy, as well as having a hysterectomy or surgical removal of the ovaries.

Everybody is unique, of course, so each woman's menopause journey will be different. Yet for many, the transition has a significant impact on their life due to a variety of physical, mental and emotional symptoms. Hopefully opening up about this midlife passage can make it easier to manage and provide some relief for what's waiting on the other side.

> *Women with menopausal symptoms can still get pregnant. Under 50s are only safe from pregnancies if they've not had a period for two years.*

HOW LONG DOES THE MENOPAUSE LAST?

The word "pause" in menopause might suggest this phase of life is just temporary. In reality, it can last a lot longer

Every woman is different, so there's no one-size-fits-all answer to this question. On average, however, the lead up to the menopause (aka the perimenopause) takes about four years. During this time women are likely to experience menopausal symptoms.

Yet once the menopause is reached (the point where periods have stopped for 12 months), symptoms can continue, on average, for another four years, as hormone levels rebalance. Different symptoms can come and go throughout this time, all varying in intensity. Plus, some women claim not to notice a thing, while others report having symptoms for up to 14 years.

Lifestyle factors, such as smoking, can influence how long the menopause lasts, and genetics also have a part to play. Symptoms vary in duration between ethnicities, too. One major study conducted in the United States discovered that black women suffer from hot flushes for a longer period of time than white women.

Symptoms

The menopause isn't just hot flushes and irregular periods – there are lots of surprising symptoms

There's a trope at play in society that depicts middle-aged women as emotional and barren beings plagued by hot flushes. Although mood changes, temperature regulation issues and a low sex drive are among the most commonly reported symptoms, these stereotypes are still dangerous.

The embarrassment women suffer coupled with an information gap on the subject of menopause means women might not discuss significant symptoms with their doctors – and there is a huge list of symptoms.

Oestrogen's role is not limited to reproduction. The hormone also has a part to play when it comes to the regulation of the central nervous system, the structure of bones and tissue, and metabolism. Cue symptoms ranging from greasy hair and dry nails to bleeding gums, brain fog, forgetfulness and weight gain.

MUSCLE ACHES AND JOINT PAINS

"An information gap means women might not discuss symptoms with their doctors"

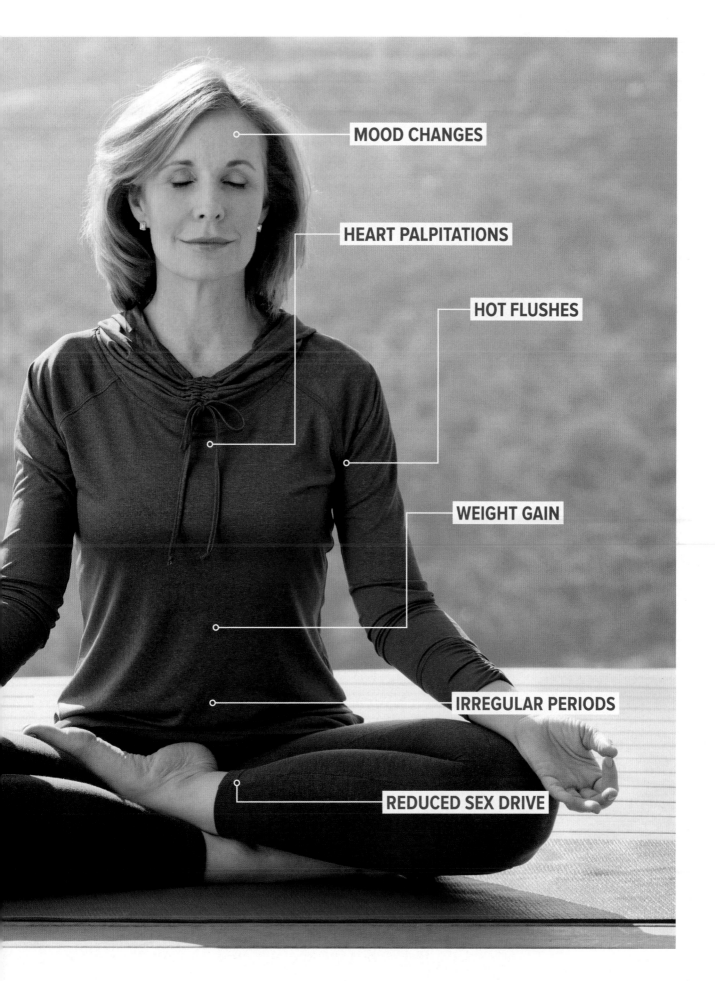

MOOD CHANGES

HEART PALPITATIONS

HOT FLUSHES

WEIGHT GAIN

IRREGULAR PERIODS

REDUCED SEX DRIVE

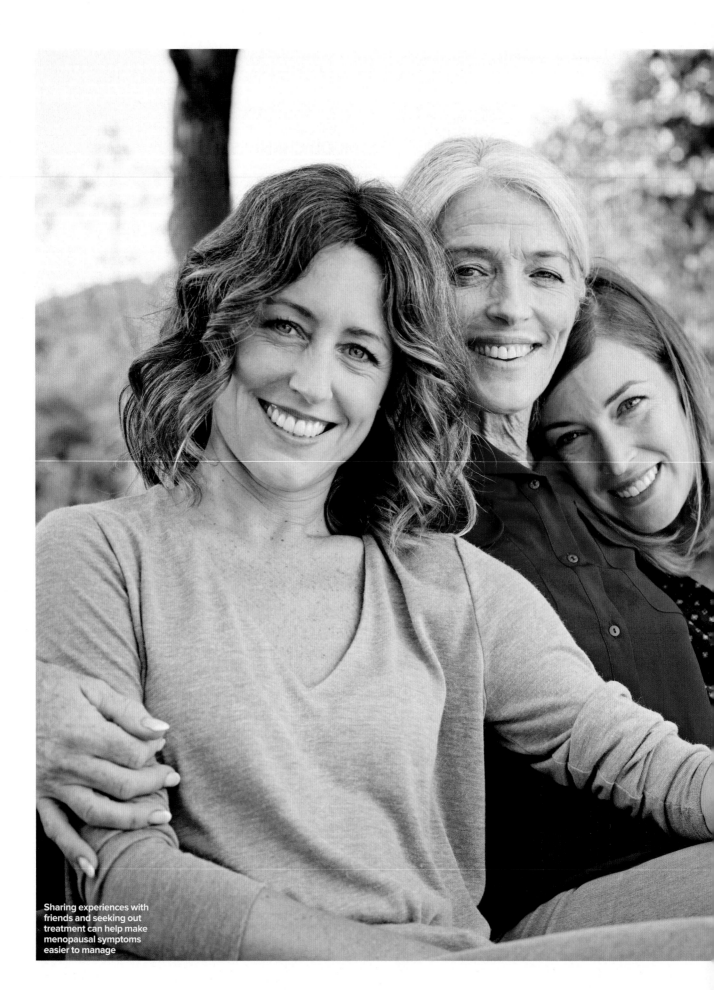

Sharing experiences with friends and seeking out treatment can help make menopausal symptoms easier to manage

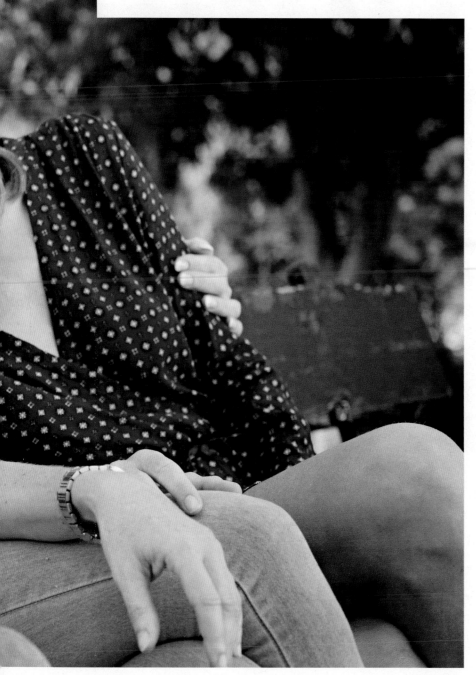

Diagnosis and
TREATMENT

Women don't have to suffer silently through the menopause, as treatments are available

When diagnosing the menopause, factors including age, symptoms and regularity of periods are taken into account. Blood tests can easily detect levels of FSH, a hormone that rises dramatically as the ovaries begin to shut down. Yet as it fluctuates throughout the perimenopause, the only way to definitely know the menopause has been reached is if a woman has not had a period for a year.

For women who seek medical help, HRT (hormone replacement therapy) is the most commonly prescribed treatment. Taken as tablets or as a patch or gel on the skin, the medication helps to relieve symptoms by replacing oestrogen levels that naturally fall in menopause.

There are some possible side effects of taking HRT, such as an increased risk of blood clots, so it's important to talk the treatment through with a medical professional. Non-hormonal treatments, including a drug called clonidine, are available too, with some women finding the relief they need in complementary therapies.

Talking therapy, CBT or anti-depressants can also be prescribed to those suffering from psychological side effects, while a testosterone replacement can help women who have lost interest in sex.

Stages

From perimenopause to postmenopause, here's what women can expect to experience

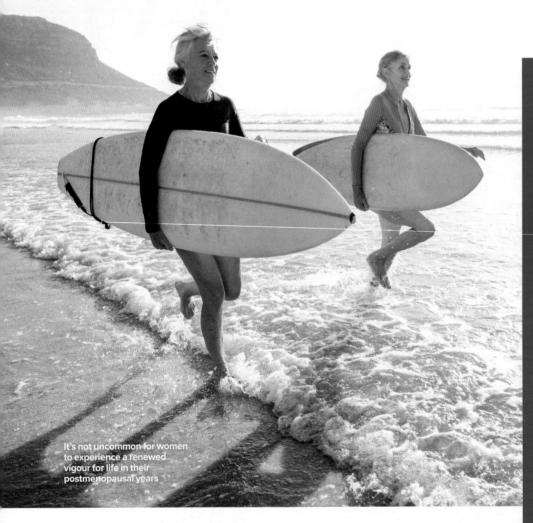

It's not uncommon for women to experience a renewed vigour for life in their postmenopausal years

MENOPAUSE IN NUMBERS

25 MILLION
women pass through menopause each year

1 in 100
women experience menopause before 40 years of age

51 is the average age periods end for good

4-8 years
Symptoms of the menopause will last on average between four and eight years

4 out of 10
women are bothered by hot flushes during the menopause

1 in 4
women say their menopause symptoms affect their quality of life

As already mentioned, the first stage of the process is known as the perimenopause. It's the period of time when ovaries gradually begin to make less oestrogen and symptoms can begin to flare up. Although associated with a decline in fertility, it's still possible to get pregnant during the perimenopause stage.

Next up is the menopause itself, the point in time when a woman has had no period for 12 consecutive months. This takes place usually between the ages of 45 and 55, and a woman is no longer able to conceive.

The final stage is the postmenopause, which continues for the rest of a woman's life. Menopausal symptoms may continue for four or so years as the body recalibrates and there are some new health concerns, including a higher risk of contracting cardiovascular disease, osteoporosis and urinary tract infections. But women generally find a renewed sense of vigour as energy levels rise and contraception is a concern of the past.

EARLY & FORCED MENOPAUSE

For some women, the menopause can make a very unexpected arrival

Words by Jo Cole

Every woman knows she will experience the menopause, with the assumption being it will occur between 45 and 55 years of age. Sometimes, though, events kick off sooner. Premature menopause starts before a woman is 40; early menopause is when it happens before she is 44. A woman can also undergo forced, or surgical, menopause as a consequence of a medical condition. While relatively rare, an understanding of what factors contribute to unexpected menopause, explored here, means those at risk can talk to their GP to discuss options.

CANCER

Radiotherapy and chemotherapy can cause a woman's ovaries to fail, resulting in forced menopause. However, it might only be a temporary menopause, and the severity depends on the type of chemotherapy, as well as which area of the body is targeted by radiotherapy. If a woman undergoes a hysterectomy or bilateral oophorectomy, it triggers immediate menopause.

NOT HAVING CHILDREN

A study by University College London and University of Queensland discovered that women who have never given birth or been pregnant are twice as likely to reach menopause before they reach 40 than those who have, and 30 percent more likely to experience early menopause. Women who have no children and who started menstruating early face a five times greater risk of premature menopause. The reasons for this are still unclear.

AUTOIMMUNE DISEASE

Premature or early menopause is a possible side effect of autoimmune disease, such as MS, rheumatoid arthritis or thyroid disease.

Autoimmune diseases cause the immune system to identify a part of the body as an enemy that needs to be attacked. This can cause inflammation, which in turn can affect the ovaries, sometimes to such an extent that it sparks the menopause.

> Smoking is shown to be a factor of early menopause. Long-term or regular smokers may experience menopause two years earlier than non-smokers.

CHROMOSOME ABNORMALITIES

A clutch of chromosome issues can affect the ovaries. For example, Turner syndrome, which the NHS says affects roughly one in 2,000 females, occurs when an X chromosome is missing or damaged. Women who have Turner syndrome might find their ovaries don't work as expected, heralding early menopause.

INFECTIONS AND BMI

Although rare, there is evidence that some infections can instigate premature or early menopause. Mumps, malaria, tuberculosis and HIV are all viruses that can affect the ovaries, leading to the menopause. The reason for this is currently unknown. Body mass can also play a part in when the menopause strikes. Oestrogen is stored in fat tissue, therefore a woman with a low BMI can't store as much, so it runs out quicker, bringing on the menopause.

TREATING EARLY MENOPAUSE
What should you do?

Although only about five percent of women experience early menopause, and one percent enter premature menopause, any menopause before the age of 45 increases the risk of osteoporosis, heart disease, strokes and type 2 diabetes. While all of these are expected health spectres of the menopause, the earlier a woman enters menopause, the more severe they can be.

Thankfully treatment is pretty standard – usually the combined contraceptive pill or hormone replacement therapy (HRT) to counteract the missing hormones, which will need to be taken until the age menopause might naturally occur, generally 51 years old.

Given the potential health consequences of early menopause, if a woman is experiencing irregular periods before she is 45, she should visit her doctor.

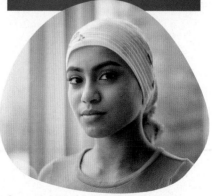

Cancer treatment can cause the menopause to happen earlier than expected, although sometimes it is a temporary state

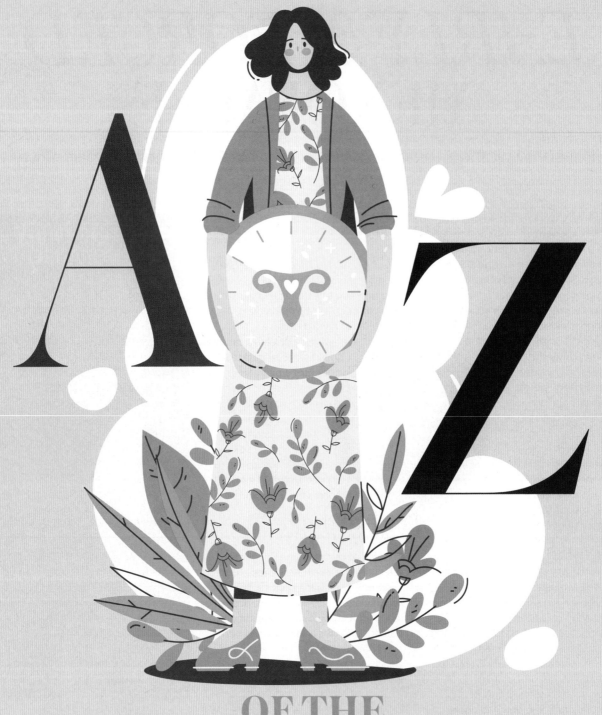

A Z
OF THE
menopause

There's more to the menopause than just hot flushes, mood changes and irregular periods, as this rundown of the side effects reveals

Words by Rebecca Bradbury

The list of menopause symptoms might be long and varied, but there's usually only one thing to blame: the duo of oestrogen and progesterone. These two hormones play a pivotal part in a woman's menstrual cycle and reproductive health. Yet in the run-up to the menopause, yo-yoing levels can cause a huge variety of physical, emotional and mental problems.

Sadly, this time of transition in a woman's life remains a taboo topic. The lack of discussion causes many to miss the connection between their symptoms and the menopause. And because each woman's journey is unique, they won't necessarily encounter all the issues discussed here. However, being able to account for the changes experienced will help make the process more manageable.

From widely-known problems such as night sweats and irritability, to surprising ailments like a dry mouth, broken fingernails and the chills, keep reading to discover the full remit of possible symptoms.

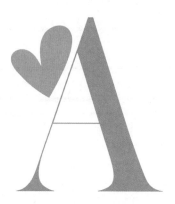

ANXIETY

Many menopausal women who experience anxiety simply think they are no longer coping like they used to. But the creeping feelings of unease, dread and foreboding, or the sudden surges of panic and fear, aren't down to age. Instead, the culprit is fluctuating hormone levels. Linking the two can help women cope with the psychological and physical symptoms, which include a fast or irregular heartbeat, shortness of breath, headaches and nausea.

Over half of those going through the menopause are said to experience mood changes, so mild anxiety is common. Frequent high levels of anxiety or panic attacks are not normal, however, and warrant a visit to the GP.

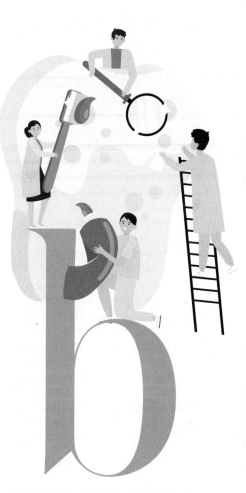

BLEEDING GUMS

Tooth trouble is one of the more unexpected symptoms of the menopause. But when you consider oestrogen is essential for healthy bones and gum tissue, it makes sense that a drop in this hormone can result in gums becoming weaker and more sensitive. Not only does this lead to bleeding gums, but it also causes conditions such as gingivitis, loose teeth and infections. At the same time, saliva production slows down, which causes a dry mouth. Not just a minor annoyance, this makes women more prone to cavities, as saliva helps defend against bacteria. Increased tooth-brushing diligence is required.

COLD FLUSHES

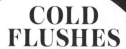

Hot flushes are almost synonymous with the menopause. Yet few realise cold flushes are a thing too. Both extremes of temperature are caused by the hypothalamus, the brain's internal thermostat, becoming overly sensitive. The body then can't regulate its temperature as efficiently. When experiencing a cold flush, the blood is being drawn away from the surface of the skin towards the internal organs, resulting in shivering and the chills. Blood vessels also get slightly less elastic due to lower oestrogen levels, which causes cold hands and feet. Some women even report feeling constantly cold while going through the menopause. Be prepared with some extra layers!

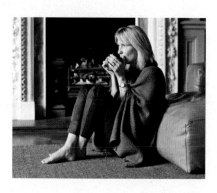

DEPRESSION

Feeling sad and melancholy is something half of all menopausal women are said to experience. Although more research is needed, the drop in oestrogen is thought to affect how the 'happy hormone' serotonin is managed. But this is not happening in isolation. Side effects of other symptoms, such as a lack of sleep, a lower sex drive and a change in body image, can also result in feeling low and unworthy. The menopause also comes at a time when parents are aging, children are leaving home and career pressure is mounting. These are all big lifestyle changes that can negatively impact stress and happiness levels, too.

Intense and prolonged feelings of sadness and recurring thoughts about death are not something to put up with. This could be clinical depression and speaking to a GP is advised.

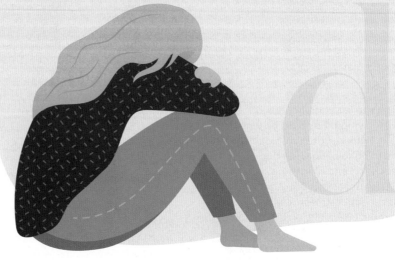

> *"The drop in oestrogen is thought to affect the 'happy hormone'"*

ELECTRIC SHOCK SENSATION (ESS)

Ever had the sensation of a rubber band snapping in the layers of tissue between the skin and muscle? Sounds strange, but for some menopausal women, it's a regular occurrence and often acts as a precursor to a hot flush. As the name suggests, the feeling is similar to getting an electric shock and it is caused by signals travelling along the central nervous system to the brain getting crossed, short-circuited or amplified. Again, it's down to oestrogen, which has a role in regulating the central nervous system. When the hormone dips, so does its ability to control signals to and from the brain.

FATIGUE

As hormone levels fluctuate, so do energy levels. Sharp drops of oestrogen results in tiredness similar to the lethargy those suffering from premenstrual tension experience. Unfortunately, menopausal women are often unable to get the sleep they so desperately need. Erratic hormone levels prevent the body from relaxing and the brain from switching off. Then there are the dreaded night sweats to contend with, which will undoubtedly make for a wakeful night. When fatigue becomes constant and severe, it can dramatically impact a person's quality of life, so sleep hygiene should be a priority for all menopausal women.

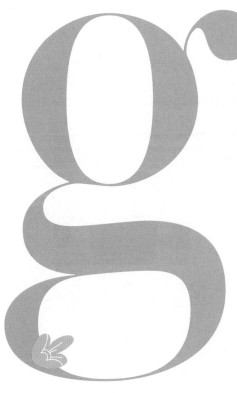

GREASY HAIR

Lank, oily hair is something both genders experience while going through puberty. So it should be no surprise that the same is experienced during another hormonal upheaval, yet it comes as a shock to many women. Menopausal changes cause surges of androgen, a hormone that increases the production of an oily lubricant called sebum in the scalp (and also the skin). As we age, hair gets thinner too, which means there is less to absorb the oil – something most teenagers don't have to put up with! It might sound counter-intuitive, but the best way to deal with greasy hair is to limit washing to just two or three times a week, otherwise sebum production will go into overdrive.

"As we age, hair gets thinner"

H

HEADACHES

Let's start with the bad news. Women who have experienced hormonal headaches before will usually find they worsen in frequency and severity while going through the menopause. But even those who were never previously bothered by headaches may start suffering from them, too.

More than half of women who suffer from migraines notice a link to their periods, so when the menopause disrupts the menstruation cycle, migraines occur more often. They are thought to happen because oestrogen controls chemicals in the brain that affect a woman's pain sensation.

Now the good news – headaches brought about by hormonal changes usually stop after the menopause.

I IRRITABILITY

Around three quarters of women describe irritability as their main emotional problem during the menopause. From becoming less tolerant and more easily annoyed, to experiencing surges of anger and rage, these psychological symptoms are caused by disruptions to the production of the mood regulator, serotonin. Women who experience similar symptoms in the run-up to their period, aka premenstrual tension, are more likely to suffer from these mood changes during the menopause, when the spikes in oestrogen are all the more dramatic.

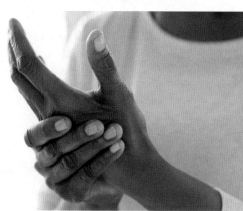

JOINT PAIN

Another symptom of the menopause that often goes under the radar is joint pain and stiffness. Although it mainly affects smaller joints, such as those in the hand, aching can also occur in the neck, shoulders and knees. Oestrogen keeps our cartilage healthy, reduces inflammation and helps with the natural replacement of bone in our body. Once this is understood, it's no shock that plummeting hormone levels can cause joints to ache and old injuries to flare up. There is also a risk of developing menopause-related osteoarthritis.

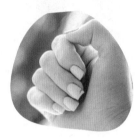

KERATIN WEAKENING

A type of protein, keratin forms the cells that make up the tissue of our nails. A drop in oestrogen, however, weakens the keratin layer so nails become brittle and break more easily. The protein is also responsible for holding the cells of our hair and skin together, with some menopausal women complaining of dull, lacklustre and thinning locks, and dry flaky skin. The likelihood of developing seborrheic keratosis, a condition that causes the skin to grow bumpy, cracked lesions, rises too.

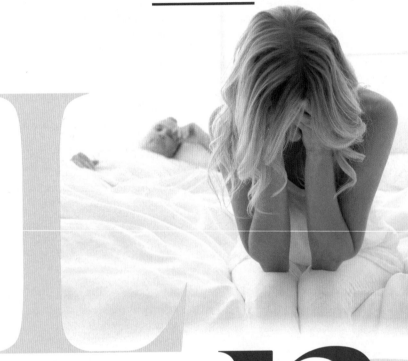

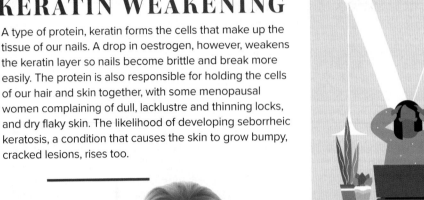

MEMORY LOSS

Feeling forgetful during the menopause can be completely normal. Research into why hormonal changes cause this cognitive issue is lacking, but experts believe it's down to oestrogen no longer being able to help the neurotransmitters involved in memory and information processing as effectively. Thankfully, once you hit the postmenopause stage, memory problems often fix themselves.

More serious symptoms, such as repeating questions or comments, getting lost in places you know well and forgetting how to use common objects, might not be down to hormonal changes. They could be a sign of dementia, in which case it's advisable to make an appointment with a GP.

LOW LIBIDO

Women are more likely than men to notice a decline in their sex drive as they age. Much of this is down to the menopause. Lower oestrogen levels dampen arousal and decrease blood flow to the vagina. This in turn causes the vaginal tissue to become thinner and less sensitive to sexual stimulation. At the same time, vaginal lubrication decreases. These changes mean women find it harder to achieve orgasm and sex may become uncomfortable or even painful. Changes in body composition can also affect a woman's self-esteem in the bedroom.

But some women begin to feel a sense of liberation. With more privacy now their children have left home and contraception no longer a consideration, libido can sometimes soar.

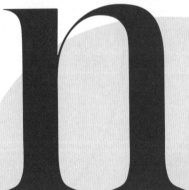

NIGHT SWEATS

Being woken up in the middle of the night due to sudden and intense flushes of warmth soaring through the body is one of the most intense symptoms of the menopause. It is also one of the most common, and regularly accompanied by excessive sweating, flushing of the neck and chest, and a racing heart. Hormonal changes are to blame once again, as the surges of oestrogen send the body's temperature control mechanism into overdrive. Not just an unpleasant experience, night sweats also prevent the sufferer from having a good night's sleep, negatively impacting the day ahead. Wearing breathable fabrics to bed, creating a cool environment to sleep in, and avoiding caffeine and spicy foods can help manage the problem.

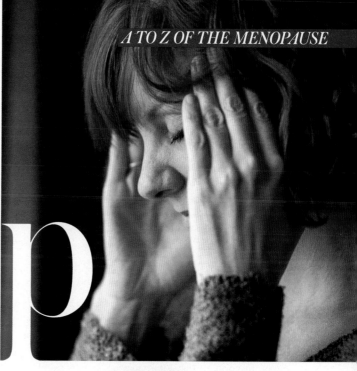

OSTEOPOROSIS

Bone strength in women begins to slowly decline from 30 years of age, speeding up significantly when the menopause hits. As oestrogen helps maintain bone health, waning levels can put women at a risk of developing osteoporosis – a condition in which bones become thin, less dense and, therefore, more likely to fracture. Those going through an early menopause (before 45 years) have a higher chance of developing osteoporosis as the normal process of declining bone density will begin earlier and continue for longer. All women are at risk though, and medical experts recommend participating in weight-bearing physical activity, maintaining a healthy weight and eating foods rich in calcium and vitamin D.

POOR CONCENTRATION

In one survey, more than half of the menopausal women questioned reported a difficulty in concentrating, as well as 'brain fog' – a symptom characterised by confusion, forgetfulness and a lack of focus and mental clarity. The disruptive effect declining oestrogen levels have on the body's neurotransmitters are thought to cause these cognitive problems – although much more research on the topic is needed. Plus, not getting enough sleep at night due to the other menopausal side effects, such as night sweats, trouble switching off and joint pain, will also impact a woman's ability to focus the next day.

"Bone strength in women begins to slowly decline from 30 years of age"

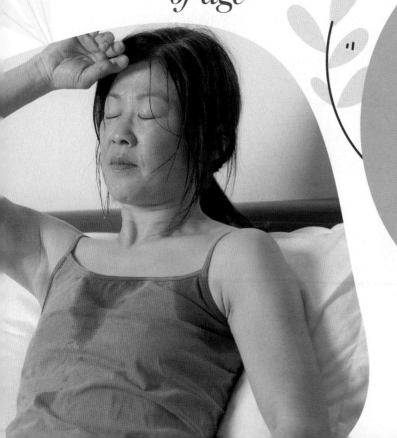

QUESTIONS

The menopause might be one of the biggest changes a woman goes through, but it still remains a huge stigma. Contributing to this problem are factors such as ageing being viewed negatively, the lack of open discussion about sexual health and the sexism still at play in society. As a result, there is not enough discourse and resources available. Research in the area, like other women's health problems, is also lacking. It's hardly surprising women have a whole host of questions concerning the menopause that they would very much like answered.

RINGING EARS

Between the ages of 20 and 69, men are almost twice as likely than women to develop hearing loss for the frequency of sounds in everyday speech. This difference between the two sexes is thought to be down to women having higher levels of oestrogen and the hormone protecting the inner ear in some way. More research is needed on the topic, but if this is the case, it explains why women who do suffer from hearing loss, usually do so around the time of their menopause. It would also provide an explanation for the ringing, roaring, hissing and other unwanted noises some menopausal women experience in their inner ear.

TENSE MUSCLES

Behind the tense, painful or cramped muscles menopausal women might experience are a number of confused hormones. Of course, oestrogen is at play again. Normally it has an inhibitive effect on the stress hormone, cortisol. Therefore, as oestrogen levels drop, the levels of cortisol rise, presenting in the body as tightened and fatigued muscles. Then there's progesterone, which has a calming effect on the body. But when levels decline, such as during the menopause, the body experiences both mental and physical symptoms of stress, including tense muscles. Suffering from other symptoms, as well as fraught lifestyle changes, can also be behind rising stress levels and the consequential stiff shoulders and clenched jaw.

SLOW METABOLISM

Oestrogen has many functions, including contributing to the operation of a woman's metabolism. Lower levels of the hormone results in a lower metabolic rate, the speed at which the body converts stored energy into working energy. This results in weight gain and, due to the effects of ageing, the fat stored in the hips and thighs will shift to the abdomen.

Studies also show that a lack of oestrogen causes the body to use starch and sugar less effectively, which again has a negative impact on the way a body metabolises energy. Such changes to the body can also impact a woman's self-esteem. Eating a well-balanced diet rich in vitamins and minerals, plus keeping as active as possible, is important to help maintain a healthy weight.

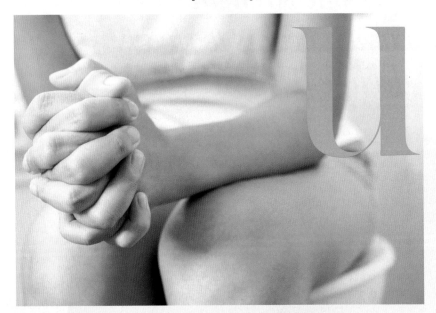

URINARY INCONTINENCE

One of the most taboo topics of the menopause is incontinence. Yet, it's completely normal for women at this time in their life to find it harder to control their bladder. Hormonal changes cause the lining of the urethra, the tube that empties urine from the bladder, to thin. Cue leaking while coughing, sneezing or laughing, as well as the sudden urge to pee and waking up in the night to use the loo more often. Women who have had a vaginal birth might struggle with this more, as their pelvic floor is at a higher risk of weakening.

VERTIGO

Dizziness is certainly not the first symptom that comes to mind when you think of the menopause, but it affects a surprisingly significant number of women. Researchers don't fully understand the connection just yet, but it's believed to be down to oestrogen and the weakening effect it has on the otoconia, an organ in the inner ear responsible for sensing the body's balance. Alternatively, vertigo could be a side effect of other menopausal symptoms, including changes to the neural system, tiredness and fatigue, and unstable blood sugar levels due to the body's decreased insulin resistance.

WATER RETENTION

Swollen ankles, puffy eyes and a bloated belly are all signs of water retention, and a common complaint among menopausal and premenstrual women. There are quite a few things going on here. Firstly, oestrogen assists with the body's regulation of water, so fluctuating levels will lead to retention. Surges of the hormone also impact the adrenal glands, responsible for producing aldosterone, a hormone that affects kidney function. This leads to imbalances between water and salt, another cause of bloating. Lastly, if oestrogen levels become much higher than progesterone, a natural diuretic, the body will hold onto more water than it should. Yet conversely, high levels of progesterone causes food to move more slowly through the intestine, again leading to bloating.

ZITS

Many hope to leave acne behind when they enter adulthood. But unfortunately spots can strike again when hormones are in flux during the menopause. While teenagers tend to suffer from breakouts on their T-zone, menopausal acne usually appears around the chin and jaw. There's also evidence to suggest those who suffered from acne in their teens may be predisposed to it again during the menopause. Breakouts are hard at any age and can understandably have a negative effect on someone's self-esteem. However, it generally tends to be a temporary condition and should disappear when hormones level out.

YEAST INFECTIONS

Most women are likely to get a yeast infection, such as vaginal thrush, at some point in their life, whether it's triggered by sex, pregnancy or antibiotics. Yet infections can occur more regularly during and after the menopause. Vaginal atrophy, where the lining of the vagina gets dryer and thinner, occurs during this time and these changes can lead to the imbalance of a women's vaginal microbiome and PH level. These conditions can cause yeast infections to develop. Symptoms include itching, swelling, redness and a white, clumpy or watery discharge.

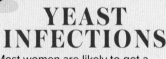

EXTREMITY TINGLING

We all know that sitting or sleeping on a body part cuts off the blood supply to the nerves and causes paraesthesia – or pins and needles as it is more commonly called. But it's a lot more alarming when a similar sense of numbness, tingling and prickling happens without an apparent cause. This is what happens to some menopausal women, generally occurring most frequently in the hands and feet. Thankfully, there is an explanation: oestrogen is affecting how the central nervous system sends its signals.

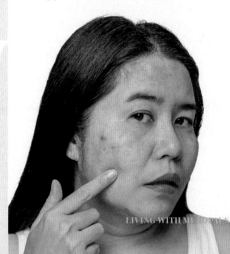

Health RISKS

As if hot flashes and mood swings weren't enough, nature has to throw a whole host of health complications into the marvelous mix that is the menopause

Words by Natalie Denton

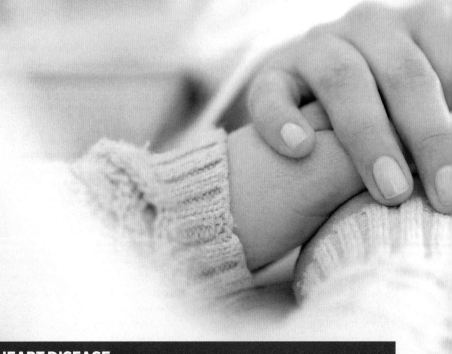

The main culprit behind the depressing string of potential health woes associated with 'the change', is the lowering levels of hormones, in particular our old vanishing friend, oestrogen. Its slow and steady disappearance from our body causes many areas to, not wanting to sugar-coat it, give up. But you're not the type of person to give up! So there are plenty of things you can do, besides taking HRT, to help your body carry on as normal. A healthy diet and regular exercise are a couple of the obvious options, but read on to find out what else you can do.

OSTEOPOROSIS

A decreasing level of oestrogen is to blame for a whole host of health woes during the menopause and afterwards too. One of the most common is osteoporosis, a condition that weakens bones, making them more vulnerable to breakages. But it's not all doom and gloom, because there are things you can do to slow its progress. Taking HRT helps, and what's more, the longer you take it the more effective it is. Keep active! Focus on weight-bearing exercises with impact (such as dancing, low-impact aerobics, even gardening) and muscle strengthening (you can use anything from a can of beans to a resistance band or weights). Consume a nutritious diet (being sure to eat healthy sources of calcium such as low-fat milk and yoghurt), plus calcium and vitamin D supplements.

HEART DISEASE

No one likes being told "no", but when it comes to looking after your heart health, this is the time in your life when no really has to mean no. No excessive indulgences, be it sugar, salt, caffeine, alcohol or cigarettes. Instead it ought to be "Yes!" to a healthy diet, full of fresh fruits and vegetables and whole foods, and yes to a healthy lifestyle, jam-packed with regular exercise and activity. The reason being, lower levels of oestrogen can cause the coronary arteries to narrow, which therefore inflates the risk of heart disease and stroke.

URINARY INCONTINENCE

Just when you thought menopause couldn't get any worse, nature throws this one your way, although regular pelvic floor exercises can help. Simply get comfy, close your eyes and focus on the muscles that stop the urine flow. Squeeze these for up to five seconds and release, then repeat ten times. Aim to do this at least three times throughout the day. Incontinency happens due to a loss of elasticity in the tissues of the urethra and vagina, making it feel like you need to 'go' when you actually don't, as well as accidentally urinating, most commonly when coughing, laughing, jumping or lifting. A lovely knockon complication of this can be more urinary tract infections (UTIs). To prevent the chance of a UTI, drink lots of water to flush out any nasty bacteria stuck in the tract, and empty your bladder as much as possible when going to the toilet.

VAGINAL DRYNESS

Not only does vaginal dryness mean being sore and itchy down there, but it can make sex feel uncomfortable and painful too, which is incredibly unhelpful when coupled with an also dimenshing sexual libido. But there are things you can use to soothe the soreness; vaginal moisturisers and unperfumed soaps are a good start. When it comes to sex, try a water-based lube for a more enjoyable experience, and focus on foreplay or use sex toys to aid natural stimulation.

HAIR THINNING

Hormonal changes are once again to blame for this confidence-crippling side effect of the menopause, because lower levels cause hair to grow at a much slower rate, therefore your tresses feel thinner as it takes longer to replace those that have naturally shed. Things that can help avoid this happening as much as possible include: relaxation (avoid stress), keep active, eat healthily (especially foods rich in fatty-acids such as almonds, walnuts, tuna and salmon), take supplements (particularly Omega-3, flavonoids and vitamins A, C, D and E), drink lots of water, and nurture your hair with a good shampoo, avoid dyes, heating devices, chlorine (use a cap) and UV rays (pop on a hat).

CANCER

Menopause doesn't cause cancer, let's just get that straight. However, there are some factors relating to the menopause which can increase the risk of some cancers, in particular, the age you are when you start the menopause. The theory behind this is that the later you start your menopause the more exposure to hormones (such as oestrogen) you'll receive, coupled with the fact you'll experience more ovulations. These two factors therefore increase the risk of breast, ovarian and uterine cancers, particularly in women who started their periods before the age of 12 and/or began menopause after 55. Cancer screenings are vital, so make sure you're seen and screened on a regular basis.

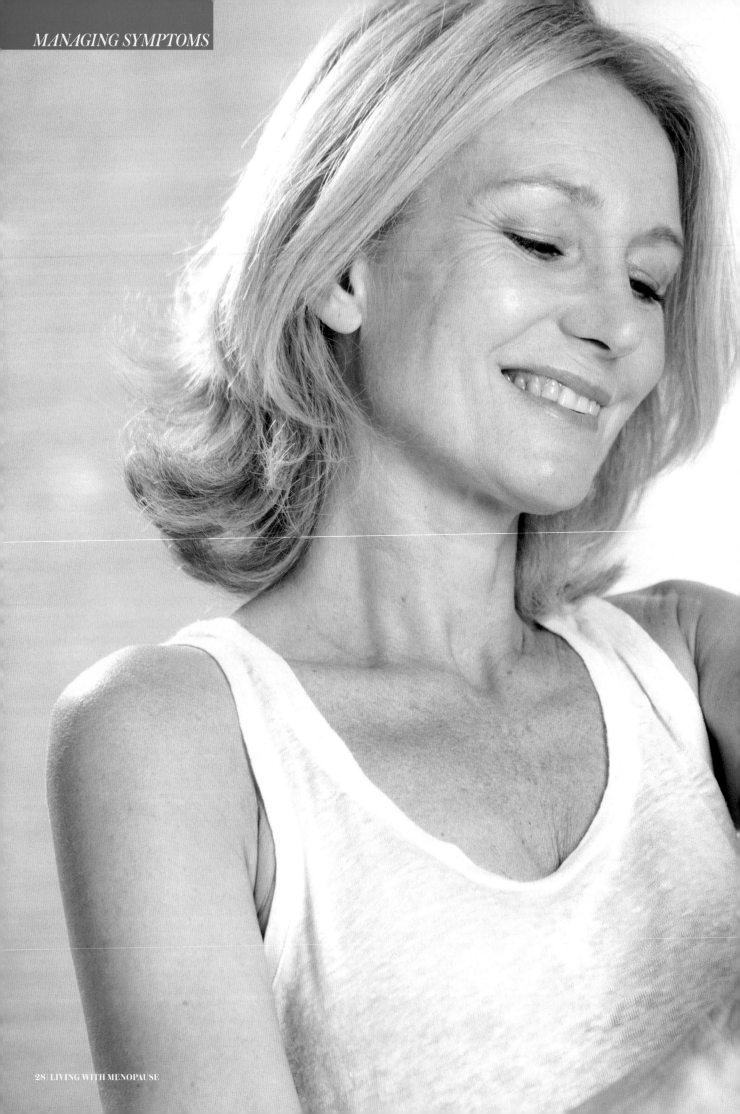

Managing your
SYMPTOMS

When life gives you lemons... how to make the most of your menopause

So you're going through the menopause. As inevitable and unrelenting as the tide, you can't stop it even if you wanted to. However, there are ways of managing your menopause to make the process less of an ordeal. There are plenty of treatments on the market to help you deal with any symptoms you may experience, from medicinal to mental. And let's not forget, you aren't in this alone. Billions of women throughout history have gone through exactly what you are right now and each has their own story to tell – some of which you'll see on the coming pages. All of this will hopefully make your menopausal journey that little bit easier.

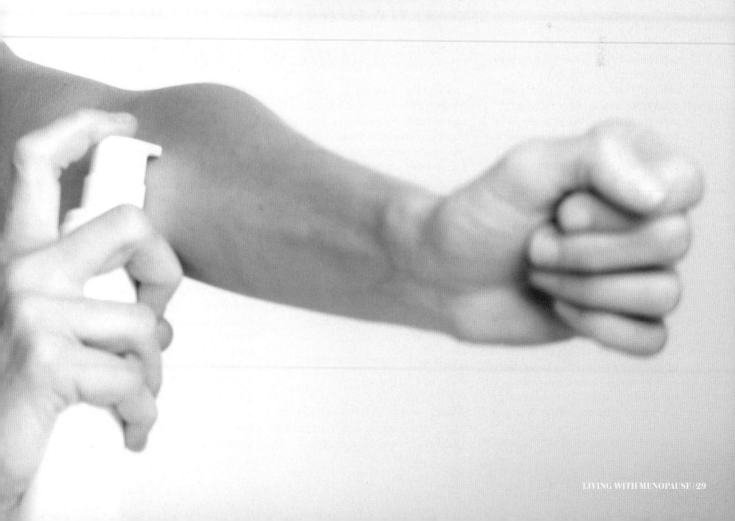

How to COPE

As with any trying time, it's okay to ask for help.
Here's a rundown of exactly how to get it...

Words by Natalie Denton

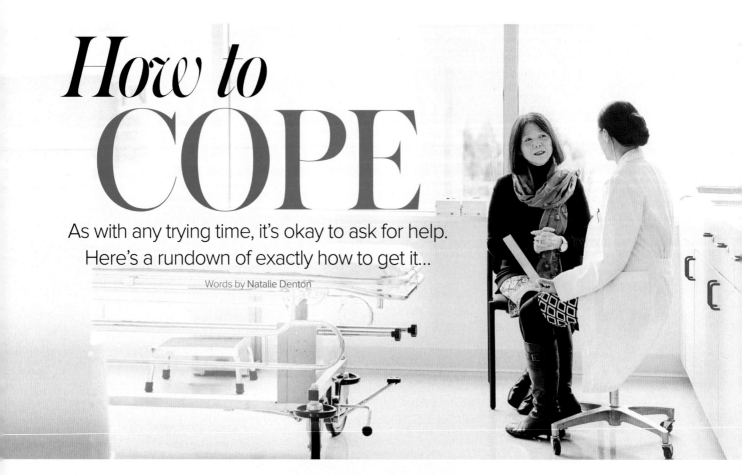

STEP 1:
Is it menopause?

With perimenopause, there is never a clear "this is happening" moment, as symptoms can begin very subtly, they come and go, you may get a few different ones sporadically and then nothing for a while. Also everyone is different, so it's not like you can compare and contrast with your female friends and relatives. It's only when your periods have stopped for 12 consecutive months that you are said to have reached menopause. But there are other reasons and health issues that can cause your periods to stop, so it's always best to check with your GP, as they can do a simple blood test to be sure.

STEP 2:
Help yourself

Waiting for your appointment can feel like torture, especially if you're desperate for medication to alleviate any symptoms you're experiencing. However, there are a number of things you can do in the meantime. First, look at making your diet more balanced, stocked full of fresh fruit, veg, healthy

"It's always best to check with your GP"

'fats' and lean proteins, as well as drinking more water and taking supplements. Increase your exercise to boost your mood, maintain a healthy weight and help combat sleep issues. If hot flushes are bothering you, opt for layers, carry a fan (the ones that spray water are a boon in the summer), and avoid triggers like caffeine, hot drinks, alcohol and spicy foods. For vaginal discomfort, there are water-based lubricants and moisturisers you can buy over the counter at a pharmacy, plus it's also been suggested that staying sexually active (thus upping the blood flow to this area) can work wonders too.

STEP 3:
Preparing to see the doctor

Visiting the doctors can be a daunting prospect for anyone, as often it can be a job to remember everything you

wanted to ask and then listen and retain all the information they tell you, with or without brain fog! So the best thing to do is write everything down, before your appointment and during it. So, after you've made that appointment, keep a logbook or journal of all the symptoms you've been experiencing, plus the day, time and how severe they were. It's a good idea to note down all the medication you take (prescribed as well as herbal and vitamin supplements) and list any relevant medical history that's affected you or your family members that could impact on what medication your doctor can recommend (for example some cancers and heart conditions).

Take a few moments to yourself to really think about what you want to get out of this appointment and write this down, followed by any and all the questions you want answers to (see opposite page for ideas).

If you're still feeling uneasy, why not ask someone to go with you to the appointment? Two heads are better than one after all!

STEP 4:
What to expect at the doctors

Once you've explained to the doctor your symptoms, or shown (and undoubtedly impressed them with) the journal you've been keeping, they may still have some questions they'll need answering before knowing how to proceed, such as:

- *Are you still having periods? If not, what was the date of your last one?*
- *On a scale of one to ten how much do each of the symptoms you are experiencing bother you?*

- *Has anything you've done or tried so far made a difference in improving any of the symptoms?*
- *Likewise, does anything make the symptoms worse?*
- *What's your diet like?*
- *How active are you?*
- *What are your stress levels like?*
- *How much alcohol and cigarettes do you consume in an average week?*

They may do a blood test or ask for a urine sample to evaluate your hormone levels, which will tell them if it is the menopause or not, and they may also check your blood pressure.

This is the time to ask the questions you've prepared, and feel free to make notes as they talk, or you could even record the conversation on your phone if they agree.

QUESTIONS TO ASK YOUR DOCTOR

Not sure what to ask at your appointment, or need a bit of inspiration? Well look no further...

- Is this definitely the menopause or could it be something else?
- *Should I have a blood test to know for sure?*
- What medication can you prescribe me to help with each of my symptoms?
- *Are these medications safe for me to take?*
- What are all the risks and/or side effects of taking them?
- *Can I drink alcohol while taking this medication?*
- How long do I need to stay on the medication for?
- *What happens if I miss a day?*
- What happens if I accidentally take/use too much?
- *How long do these symptoms typically last for?*
- Will these symptoms ever go away or are they permanent?
- *Do I need to book a follow-up appointment(s)? If so, when/how regularly?*
- Do I need to have regular blood tests?
- *Other than medication,*

what else can I do to help alleviate my symptoms?
- Are there any alternative therapies or medications you can recommend?
- *How will my future health be impacted?*
- What can I do to help myself in terms of staying as healthy as possible, for as long as possible?
- *Is there anywhere I can read further information about what's happening to me, either on a pamphlet, website, book or app?*
- Can you recommend any support groups or helplines?

STEP 5:
After the doctors

Hopefully you should leave your appointment feeling relieved and better informed, as the doctor should have answered your questions and eased your fears. They should also have explained: the stages of menopause, other possible symptoms, suggested lifestyle changes to improve your wellbeing, outlined all the medication available to you as well as the risks of treatment, how your future health could be affected, and what you can do to help yourself.

If you have been prescribed medication it's worth keeping a note somewhere (on your phone, or maybe on the fridge) of what you need to take, when, how much and how often. A weekly pill organiser, with the days of the week on the lid, can be a great way to stay organised and ensure you take what you need, when you need it.

Continue with your symptoms journal, noting if things are improving or worsening. If it's the latter, be sure to make a follow-up appointment with your doctor to evaluate.

STEP 6:
Find help in all the right places

Once you've seen the doctor, started taking the medication and adjusted your lifestyle you may be left wondering what's next. Why not try a new sport or activity? Not only will this help with your symptoms but it'll improve your health in many ways and give you the opportunity to meet new people, perhaps other women who are going through the same thing. What's more, this will give you the chance to talk about how you're feeling. There are menopause specific support groups out there too. Just look online to find one near to where you are, or arrange to spend time with friends and family to open up about what exactly you have been going through.

Menopause is such a big change – emotionally and physically – and it's important you feel supported and loved. So be kind to yourself, acknowledge what you're going through and give yourself credit for everything you're overcoming.

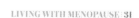

12 Menopause MYTHS BUSTED!

From misinformation around HRT to doom-ladened advice about your sex life, the menopause is a hot topic for gossip. We sift fact from fiction...

Words by **Sophie Barton**

1 I CAN'T GET PREGNANT

If you're considering ditching contraception, you need to think again! "It's recommended that you use contraception for two years after your last menstrual period, as a random ovulation can occur," says Dr Ghazala Aziz-Scott from the Marion Gluck Clinic (**mariongluckclinic. com**). "There can be a last-ditch attempt by the body to get pregnant before ovulation totally ceases."

2 IT BEGINS AT 50

The average UK age for the menopause – when periods have stopped for 12 months – is 51. However, the perimenopausal period typically begins from the mid 40s. "During the perimenopausal period, periods become more erratic and hormone levels fluctuate, causing symptoms like hot flushes and insomnia," says Dr Aziz-Scott.

3 I'LL HAVE WEAK BONES

Bone density does decline throughout the menopause, but this can be addressed. Dr Aziz-Scott says: "HRT (hormone replacement therapy), a healthy diet with a good intake of calcium and vitamin D, a good bone supplement and plenty of weight bearing exercise can help keep your bones strong and robust."

4 HOT FLUSHES ARE THE FIRST SYMPTOM

Hot flushes are often talked about, but may not be the first symptom. This is "often anxiety and insomnia, which are symptoms of progesterone deficiency," explains Dr Aziz-Scott. "Cognitive changes such as brain fog and memory loss are also common."

5 I'LL GAIN WEIGHT

Hormonal changes can result in a slowing metabolism, making it harder to maintain your weight. But it's not all bad news. Dr Aziz-Scott says: "A healthy lifestyle with a Mediterranean-style diet and good levels of movement and exercise can go a long way towards mitigating weight gain."

6 MY SEX LIFE IS OVER

Changes in oestrogen and testosterone can dampen your libido and trigger vaginal dryness, but don't despair. Dr Ghazala Aziz-Scott says: "With adequate hormone replacement and vaginal oestrogen, your love life can be restored." Vaginal oestrogen is low-dose oestrogen, which is applied directly inside the vagina to help rebuild the lining and promote lubrication.

7 HRT IS THE ONLY SOLUTION

HRT can have great benefits, including improved cardiovascular health and the prevention of osteoporosis and dementia, but lifestyle changes help too. Dr Aziz-Scott says: "There are natural ways of handling this phase of life, including resistance training, stress reduction, ensuring good sleep and supplements like omega-3 fish oils and magnesium."

8 IT'S ALWAYS TOUGH

It's human nature to focus on the negatives surrounding the menopause, but it's not all doom and gloom – not everyone struggles. "Many women do sail through this period," adds Dr Aziz-Scott.

9 LATER PUBERTY MEANS LATER MENOPAUSE

Dr Aziz-Scott thinks there is unlikely to be a direct link between when you started your period and when you begin the perimenopause. However, studies suggest that if your mum went through it early, you might do the same. She adds: "There may be some genetic element, especially if there's a family history of premature menopause."

"HRT can have great benefits, but lifestyle changes help too"

10 THE SYMPTOMS ARE JUST PHYSICAL

We know about irregular periods and hot flushes, but changing hormones will probably affect our emotions too. Dr Aziz-Scott says: "Progesterone is our natural calming hormone, so anxiety and mood changes are very common. Oestrogen is also linked to serotonin, our feel-good neurotransmitter, while dopamine links with testosterone and can impact motivation."

11 EVERYONE CAN TAKE HRT

HRT can have many positives, but it isn't for everyone, especially if you've experienced certain medical conditions. "Not all women can or wish to take HRT," says Dr Aziz-Scott. "It may not be safe to take if you have had breast cancer or a stroke for example." If this is the case, alternatives may be recommended.

12 IT'S DOWNHILL FROM HERE

"Life after the menopause can actually be very liberating," says Dr Aziz-Scott. "Children have flown the nest and there's more time for hobbies and leisure. It is important to maintain a positive attitude." Remember that post menopause, many of the more bothersome symptoms will fade too.

◆ **Dr Ghazala Aziz-Scott** *is a specialist in integrative women's health and bioidentical hormone balancing for the Marion Gluck Clinic, the UK's leading medical clinic that pioneered the use of bioidentical hormones to treat menopause, perimenopause and other hormone-related issues.*
www.mariongluckclinic.com

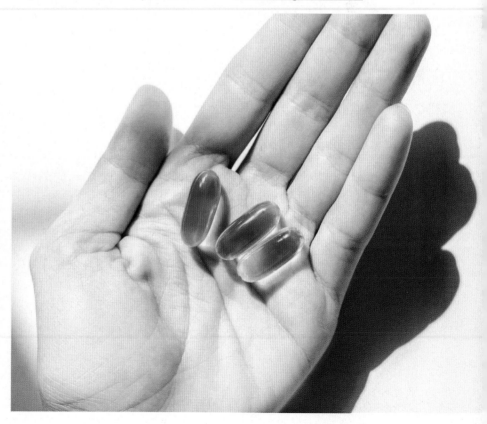

MENO

Dos

DO
TAKE A CALCIUM SUPPLEMENT

Increase bone density and protect against osteoporosis with a calcium supplement. Dr Harper, from the Harper Clinic in Harley Street, says: "Women up to age 50 need around 1,000 milligrams daily and women over 50 should aim for 1,200 milligrams daily."

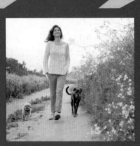

DO
KEEP MOVING

Look after mind and body with exercise. "Start with at least ten minutes a day of brisk walking," says Dr Harper. "Then, introduce strength training. It can reduce body fat, strengthen muscles and help burn calories more efficiently."

DO
TRY INTERMITTENT FASTING

If you've gained weight, aim to reduce your calorie intake. "Try intermittent fasting, which can be beneficial," suggests Dr Harper. "Don't beat yourself up about weight though, as long as you're not falling into the obesity category."

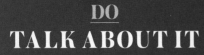

DO
AVOID CAFFEINE

Tweak your diet, to help reduce uncomfortable hot flushes. "Try to avoid caffeine, alcohol and spicy food," says Dr Harper. "Some retailers sell cooling duvets, to help during the menopause."

DO
TALK ABOUT IT

Confiding in others can help you feel as though you aren't alone. Dr Harper says: "There are some brilliant support groups out there, like Issviva (**www. issviva.com**), a free website where you can learn about menopause and share your experience."

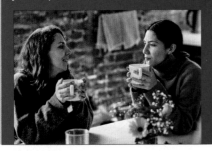

DO
BOOST YOUR BRAIN

Brain fog can be frustrating, but you can support your grey matter. "Quality sleep is key, and do consider HRT – boosting oestrogen levels helps brain connectivity," says Dr Harper. "Eat plenty of omega-3 fatty acids too, like salmon and leafy green veg."

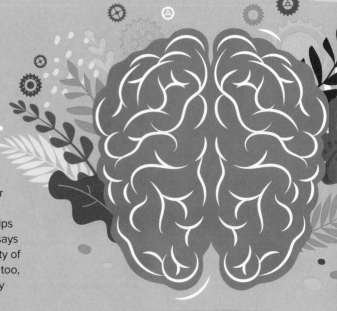

PAUSE

DON'T
BE AFRAID OF HRT

HRT doesn't just reduce the symptoms, it also reduces the risk of osteoporosis, heart disease, colon cancer and dementia. "Scare stories are based on old data, which isn't correct," says Dr Harper. "For most women, there are many more benefits than risks."

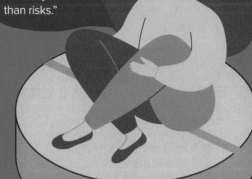

DON'T
SUFFER IN SILENCE

If your GP isn't helping, ask to see someone else. Dr Harper says: "Make a list of your symptoms or download a symptom checker. Fill it out and see whoever in your practice is most well versed in menopause." You'll find a handy symptom checker at **issviva.co.uk/test**.

DON'T
NEGLECT YOUR SKIN

During the perimenopause and menopause, we lose around 30% of our skin collagen, leading to dry skin and wrinkles. Protect skin with daily sunscreen and hydrate with moisturiser too. "A quality collagen supplement can help restore lost volume and promote skin laxity," adds Dr Harper.

Don'ts

The menopause can be a minefield to navigate. Expert Dr Shahzadi Harper guides you through what to do — and what not to do...

Words by Sophie Barton

◆ **Dr Harper** is a menopause expert from The Harper Clinic and co-author of The Perimenopause Solution. She is also an ambassador for new menopause platform, **issviva.com**

DON'T
EAT JUNK

During the menopause, your body struggles to process sugary, processed foods. "Try to consume foods that fall into the Mediterranean diet instead," says Dr Harper. This includes olive oil, nuts, seeds, avocado and fish.

DON'T
PANIC ABOUT LOW MOOD

Mental symptoms, like mood swings and anxiety, are very normal and there are treatments that can help, including HRT, cognitive behavioural therapy and mindfulness. "Explain how you feel to your GP," says Dr Harper. "Ask them to take your bloods to see if your hormone levels are normal."

DON'T
GIVE UP ON SLEEP

Night sweats and anxiety can make shut-eye a struggle, so focus on sleep hygiene. "Silk nightwear can help control your body temperature," says Dr Harper. "Don't take your phone to bed, don't drink caffeine late on and try breathing exercises to slow down your body."

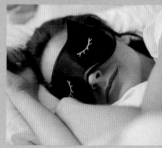

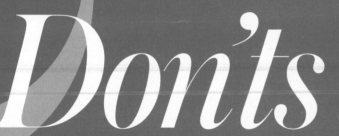

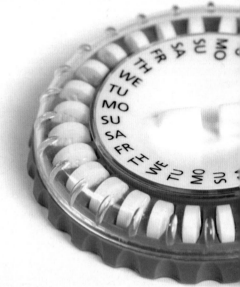

Treating
MENOPAUSE

Don't suffer unnecessarily! There are plenty of ways you can treat the symptoms of menopause...

Words by Natalie Denton

The menopause, with its cohort of menacing symptoms – be it mood swings and vaginal dryness, or night sweats and brain fog – doesn't need to be the big bad wolf it was once considered to be. Today, there are a whole host of things you can do and take to alleviate all the bother this 'time in life' can throw your way. What's more, it's not all hormone replacement drugs and medications, although these will do the trick. There are also natural alternatives, psychotherapy for mental, as well as physical problems, and then there's that age-old cure-all – exercise and activity. So don't throw the towel in just yet, or suffer in silence. Make an appointment with your medical professional and ask to fully explore all the options available to you. Be sure to detail all the symptoms you've been experiencing and divulge your medical history, as well as that of your ancestors if relevant (for example cancers and heart disease), in case this impacts the choices available to you, thus prompting your doctor to propose a series of satisfying alternatives.

TESTOSTERONE GEL

For those with a flagging sex drive, a doctor may recommend testosterone gel, which is claimed to not only bolster your libido but your mood and energy levels too. Typically it's prescribed postmenopause to those seeking to restore their sex drive, but it can be taken at the same time as HRT. Side effects are uncommon but include unwanted hair growth and acne.

VAGINAL OESTROGEN

If you've noticed your vagina feels drier than it did before, or painful or itchy, it might not be a yeast infection, but rather another delightful symptom of the menopause. Good news though. Your doctor can prescribe an oestrogen treatment that's inserted straight inside your vagina, either as a cream, tablet or ring, and can be used for the rest of your life should you want to, as rather than infiltrating your bloodstream, its work is isolated to the area it finds itself. This treatment is also said to improve other menopausal symptoms, like pain when urinating.

HORMONE REPLACEMENT THERAPY (HRT)

Effective and safe for most women, HRT can be started as soon as perimenopause commences or during any stage of the menopause. It's administered in a variety of forms including skin patch, gel, spray, implant or tablet, and works by replacing your body's lowering levels of oestrogen. In addition to oestrogen, those who have a womb will often be prescribed progesterone as well, to protect the womb's lining from the effects of taking oestrogen. Combined HRT, as it is known, can be delivered via a patch, IUS (intrauterine system or coil), or tablets.

The upside of HRT is that it combats most menopausal symptoms relatively quickly, such as brain fog, hot flushes, mood swings, vaginal dryness and joint aches. What's more, your risk of developing osteoporosis and heart disease is also said to decrease. However, as with any medications there are risks, but these are said to be small and are often outweighed by the benefits.

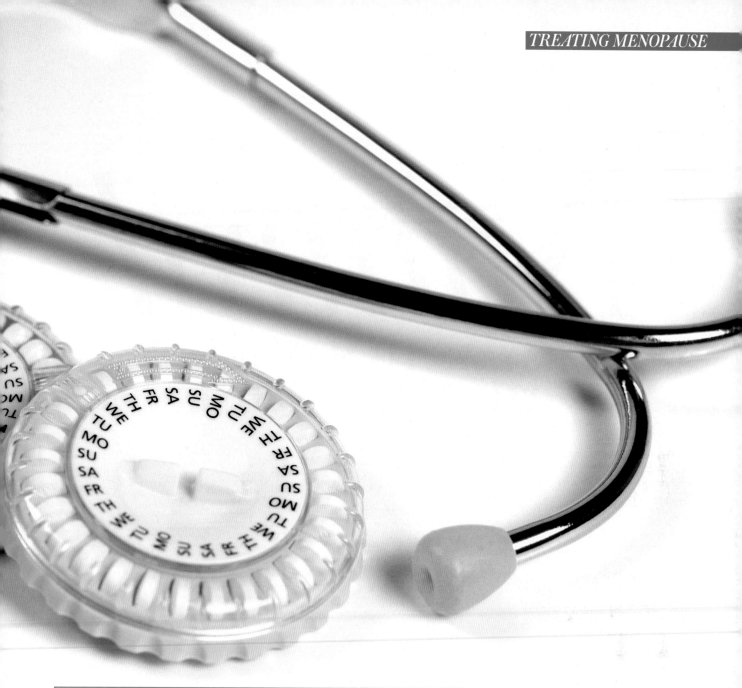

COGNITIVE BEHAVIOURAL THERAPY (CBT)

If you'd like an alternative to medication to combat changing moods, then Cognitive Behavioural Therapy (CBT) is a really productive alternative. It's thought to be able to help with some physical symptoms as well, such as joint pain and hot flushes. This can be carried out as one-on-ones or if you are feeling social, as group therapy.

NON-HORMONE MEDICINES

If you decide hormone replacement treatments aren't the way to go, there are still many other things you can do to alleviate some of the symptoms associated with the perimenopause and menopause. For starters, there is a bounty of natural alternatives, see page 38 for more on these, or a doctor can prescribe you a range of non-hormone treatments. For example, clonidine is a blood pressure medicine given to those suffering with night sweats and hot flushes, taken in tablet form twice, or sometimes three times, a day. Unlike HRT, clonidine won't affect hormone levels and therefore does not carry an increased risk of problems such as breast cancer, as can be the case with HRT. Gabapentin, a medicine traditionally used to treat epilepsy, is another viable non-hormone treatment doctors can offer menopausal women.

ANTIDEPRESSANTS

In recent years the stigma of antidepressants has mercifully dispersed, with the focus on mental health shifting from one of judgement, to one of genuine concern and care. It could be that you feel your moods are all over the place or perhaps you feel overly sensitive and irritable. It might be that you feel increasingly anxious or maybe you've been feeling low for a while. Whatever it is, it's important you talk to your doctor – just as you would if you had an ailment of the body – and ensure you get the right medication for you.

Natural

WAYS TO MANAGE YOUR MENOPAUSE

The self-care tips, tricks and remedies
to help you through the change

Words by Jane Druker

"The average age for a woman to be through her menopause is 52 [in the UK]," explains Emma Bardwell, registered nutritionist and author of *The Perimenopause Solution*. The lead-up to actual menopause – when you have not had a period for 12 consecutive months – is the perimenopause and can last for up to a decade. So, in your 40s and 50s, it can be helpful to aid the transformation of your body with physical, nutritional and self-care building blocks.

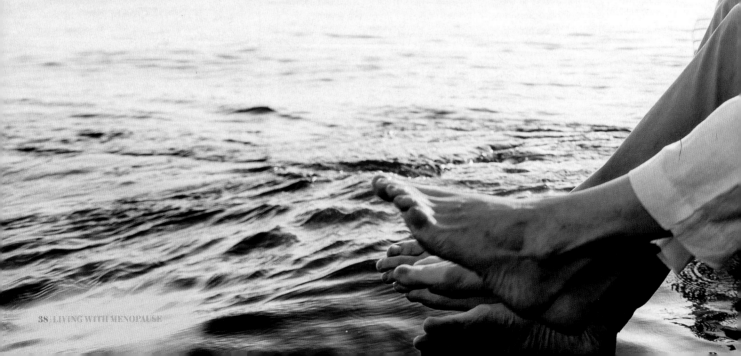

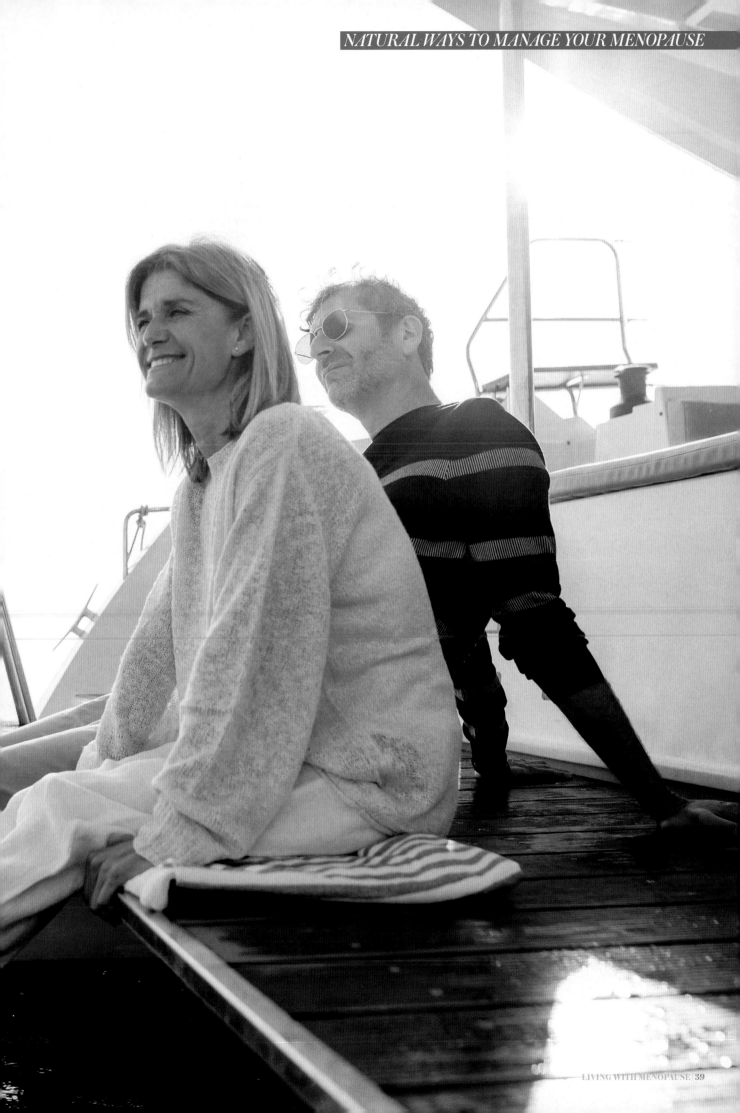

POSITIVE THINKING

"Make this time positive," says Emma. "After all, you are done with the pain and headache of having monthly periods and that crazy time in life when you are juggling it all." Instead take the opportunity to redefine yourself and think about what you like and how you want to spend your time. Self-reflection and self-congratulation are now the order of the day. You got here. Now what are you going to do with this one wild and precious life?

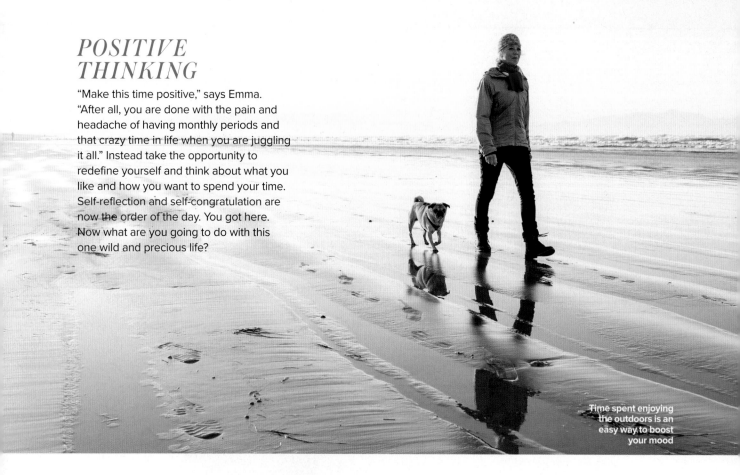

Time spent enjoying the outdoors is an easy way to boost your mood

SLEEP

"In midlife your progesterone and oestrogen hormones take a dip," explains Emma, "and that is often when the sleep issues begin". Oestrogen plays an important role in regulating melatonin production, which is responsible for sleeping patterns. A lack of it can also result in night sweats. But that's not all. "What is often overlooked is that the oestrogen receptors are in our nerve endings so women experience bladder issues, joint paint, restless leg syndrome, pins and needles and even tinnitus," adds Emma. Natural remedies are in iron and magnesium, so get your doctor to check if you have a deficiency and take supplements if needed. "Also get into a healthy daily routine – exercise, daylight and fresh air all build up the body's need to sleep – and minimise blue light in the evenings."

"Get into a healthy routine"

Take iron and magnesium for a restful slumber

SUPPLEMENTS

"There can be an overreliance on supplements," cautions Emma. "They can never replace a good diet." She recommends a calcium-rich diet of oily fish two times a week for omega-3, which is responsible for making the hormones that regulate the relaxation of the artery walls and inflammation. Sardines and pilchards are great sources because the fish bones are nutrient-dense. If you are vegetarian or vegan, all green vegetables, tofu, seeds and almonds provide this. She also recommends drinking a fortified plant milk instead of the usual dairy version.

When it comes to vitamins B and D, supplements are best as they are hard to absorb from food alone. "The B vitamins are good for hormone production and mood and vitamin D is needed for bone health and immunity." And if you need extra support, there are MenoSerene tablets, which include plant oestrogens.

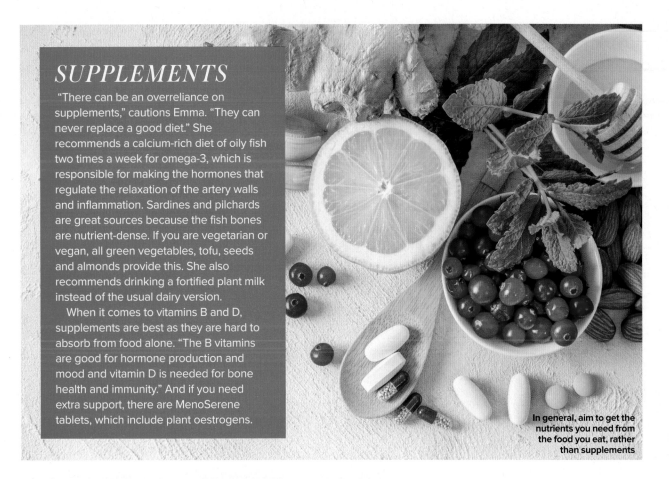

In general, aim to get the nutrients you need from the food you eat, rather than supplements

The right diet could help tackle mood swings, hot flushes and palpitations

A HEALTHY DIET

"Keeping blood sugar levels regulated is important for both anxiety and mood," explains Emma. "When it dips it puts your body into an emergency red alert state, which can bring on hot flushes and palpitations." Try eating a diet high in soya-based products and protein, which level off blood sugar, fill you up and are low in calories. Have a palm-sized piece of protein with each of your three meals. Poultry, fish and eggs are good for both their nutritional value and muscle mass. Add linseeds and flaxseeds to porridge and eat a diet rich in chickpeas, lentils and the legume family, which are full of natural phytoestrogens. "The Mediterranean diet is also known to be anti-inflammatory," adds Emma. "There is a focus on eating plants and getting a lot of fibre, so take a leaf out of the Italians' book and a good rule to follow is to eat the rainbow." She recommends a simple daily menu could look something like a breakfast of Greek yoghurt with berries and seeds and honey, lunch of omelette and salad and then a dinner of salmon and prawns with buckwheat noodles.

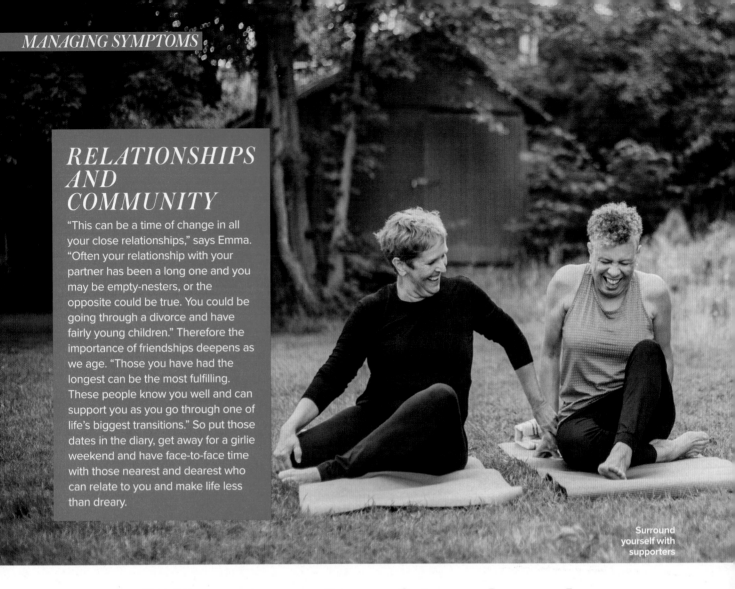

RELATIONSHIPS AND COMMUNITY

"This can be a time of change in all your close relationships," says Emma. "Often your relationship with your partner has been a long one and you may be empty-nesters, or the opposite could be true. You could be going through a divorce and have fairly young children." Therefore the importance of friendships deepens as we age. "Those you have had the longest can be the most fulfilling. These people know you well and can support you as you go through one of life's biggest transitions." So put those dates in the diary, get away for a girlie weekend and have face-to-face time with those nearest and dearest who can relate to you and make life less than dreary.

Surround yourself with supporters

"Weave in pockets of time throughout your day to do things you value"

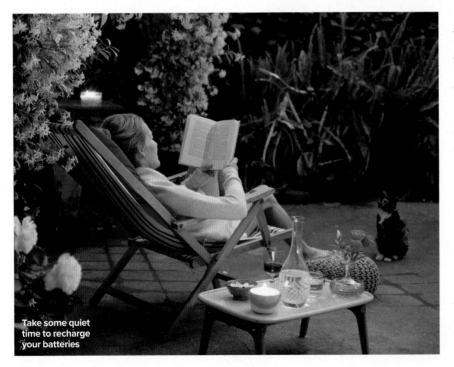

Take some quiet time to recharge your batteries

RELAX AND DE-STRESS

"Women spread themselves too thin," thinks Emma. "The perimenopause and menopause are a stark reminder to look after you." Weave in pockets of time throughout your day to listen to apps or podcasts, go for a long walk alone or with company and do things you value. "It's all part of self-care, and I also recommend learning to say no to things that do not give you joy." Both CBD and acupuncture can help to relieve anxiety and continual practice of meditation can also be helpful. "Give yourself those moments of peace and tranquility," she urges. "It's putting fuel back in the tank."

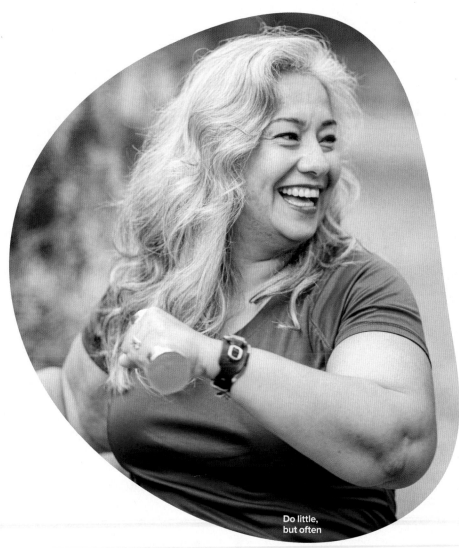

Do little, but often

EXERCISE

"Exercise is a must-do whether you are on HRT or not," explains Kate Oakley, @yourfuturefit, who became a personal trainer at 50 and specialises in training menopausal women. "But it's absolutely not about doing giant intimidating workouts. It's about doing a little often, something over nothing." A simple starting point is while you are brushing your teeth. For those two minutes, do a squat at the same time – this will have you moving your body 28 minutes a week. Or start with walking, which "is underrated for both physical and mental health", Kate says, adding "20 minutes is fine."

Build on this as and when you can; maybe start with a short six-minute resistance training programme that is slow, controlled and mindful, using a pair of dumbbells (3kg is usually a good starting point) or resistance bands. "This technique builds strength, flexibility and agility and you will get small achievable wins that will build you up to success," says Kate. In addition, it is great for your bone health – osteoporosis is a real threat of the menopause. It's also important to have a leaner muscle mass, as this is when you burn more calories even at rest, so is great for weight management.

However, take care to not go too hard on yourself. "Things like HIIT classes are good for power and heart health but if you put your body under too much stress, you end up storing the stress hormone cortisol as fat," Kate explains. Also try working out with a friend, either on FaceTime or in person. "Having an accountability buddy is a really good way of sticking with exercise as you don't want to let a friend down," says Kate. Cold water swimming is also having a moment in the sun as it tends to be done in sociable groups and helps your breathing into the bargain.

5 ESSENTIAL OILS FOR MENOPAUSE

Some essential oils contain phytoestrogens, which work in a similar way to oestrogen. Phytoestrogens aid the balance of hormones and relieve symptoms such as mood changes and hot flushes during menopause. There are various discussions about which oils are the most beneficial to menopausal women, but the five below are known to decrease body temperature and help gain some all-important equilibrium.

CLARY SAGE

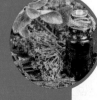

Clary sage has a similar effect on the body to oestrogen. Apply drops of the oil to the soles of your feet to help reduce hot flushes.

PEPPERMINT

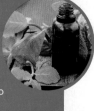

Peppermint oil can relieve pain from headaches and help with hot flushes and fatigue. Add a few drops to a tissue and breathe it in.

GERANIUM

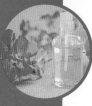

Add geranium oil to a bath to help balance out your hormones, lift your mood and heal dry skin.

BASIL

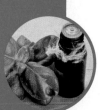

If you're tired and experiencing hot flushes, dab some basil oil on the back of your neck for a bit of relief.

LAVENDER

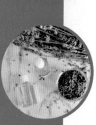

If you're anxious or losing sleep, lavender can help soothe you and reduce the effects of hot flushes, night sweats and depression.

Images: Getty

IS IT A
Big deal?

Menopause can be challenging for some women, requiring huge adjustment and medical help, while others have minimal symptoms

Words by Joan McFadden

Kirsty Wark started a big conversation with her 2017 documentary, *My Menopause and Me*, a complete eye-opener for thousands of viewers. She asked why menopause is such a loaded word, when 'the change' is a fact of life for all women, often in midlife when they're at the top of their game. Confident, articulate, experienced women too often find themselves floundering as they reach perimenopause and menopause, with lack of information and support a big problem. Now, as more women share their experiences, it's clear that menopause is different for everyone and we need to keep talking about it.

"Once we control the symptoms, we're unstoppable"

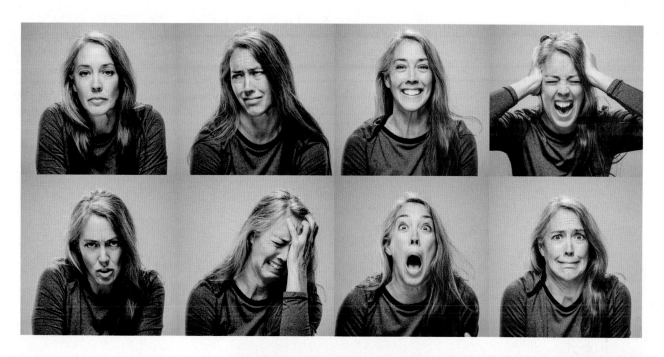

WORK WOES

Tess Caven (57) from Essex is the co-founder of a start-up walking for charity app (**www.trundl.co.uk**). "A well-woman check-up at 50 indicated I was early peri and symptoms suddenly kicked in at 52," she says. "I'm an agile thinker and drawing blanks was horrible as I worked in the creative industries. Anxiety exacerbated the problem and brought on depression. I started to get hot flushes, super embarrassing in an industry that adores the young and deems 50 an effective sell-by date for women, but wasn't just going to 'ride it out'. HRT gel got my brain back and the flushes disappeared."

Tess advises that being healthy is a good way of tackling symptoms. "I'm really well and have good levels of energy thanks to lots of walking, testing the trundl app. Don't write off taking HRT or other intervention but you have to take care of your body, find physical activities you love, check you're eating well and supplement with bone and joint support early on as a preventative measure. 'Queenager' is a good name for this time of life – once we control the symptoms, we're unstoppable."

BEGGING FOR HELP

Hyacinth Myers (50) from Hackney, is a life strategist, coach and author (**hyacinthmyers.com**). She experienced a GP who offered no help. "I was 42 when perimenopause started with night sweats, repeated urine infections, tiredness, brain fog and vaginal dryness," she says. "The GP was very dismissive, fixated on sexual health and refused a hormone test. I was finally referred to a Uro-Gynae clinic after four years of constantly asking, and after two hours they told me I was quite clearly in advanced perimenopause and why hadn't I come sooner as I now had vaginal atrophy. I was prescribed an oestrogen cream, which reversed everything and I'm alarmed that so many women feel they just have to put up with it and aren't getting the help available."

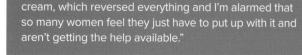

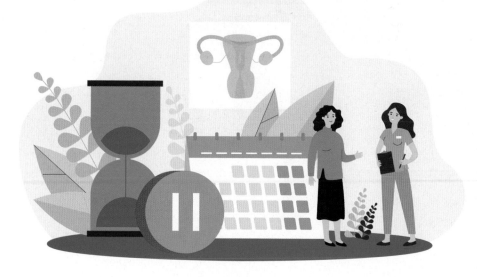

THROWN INTO MENOPAUSE

Dani Binnington (43) from Surrey is a patient's advocate for women in menopause after cancer and runs a yoga school and podcast (**healthywholeme.com**). "I was thrown into menopause at 39 after surgery to remove my ovaries, after breast cancer at 33," she says. "It's really important to plan for 'after care' when someone enters menopause through surgery or medication. Sadly, most women I speak to say they've had very little help and I want to bridge the gap.

"Managing menopause after cancer is a totally different ball game," she explains. "We must talk through our options with a specialist team to help come up with a plan for a good quality of life and long-term health too. I won't stop talking about menopause and cancer until more women are supported and heard."

LIFE CHANGES MADE MENOPAUSE EASIER

Anne Larchy (50), a weight loss and healthy lifestyle coach from Finchley, believes she inadvertently helped herself have a better menopause through earlier life changes. "Age 43 I came off the pill after a breakup with my partner," she says. "My period never came back. Six months later I went to my GP and my blood results were off the chart past the menopause. I had no symptoms so we decided against HRT and seven years later the only change is if I drink too much or eat too much sugar later in the evening and wake up, I can't sleep again."

Twelve years ago, starting as a coach, she cut out junk food, sweets, alcohol and cakes. "That's probably made my menopause easier without being aware of it, and I'm super happy I don't have to think about my period anymore."

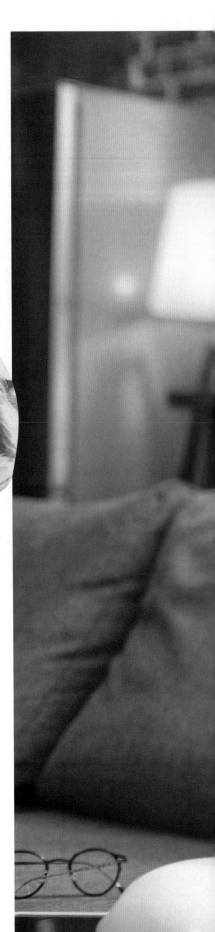

"Every woman can have a different experience"

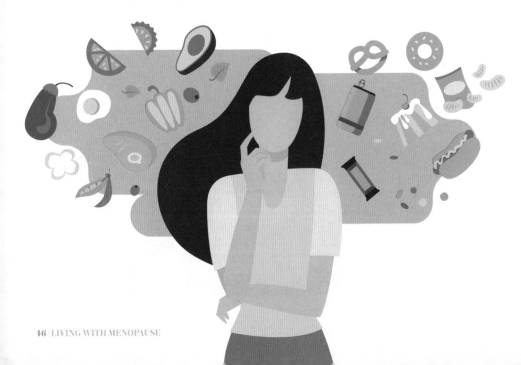

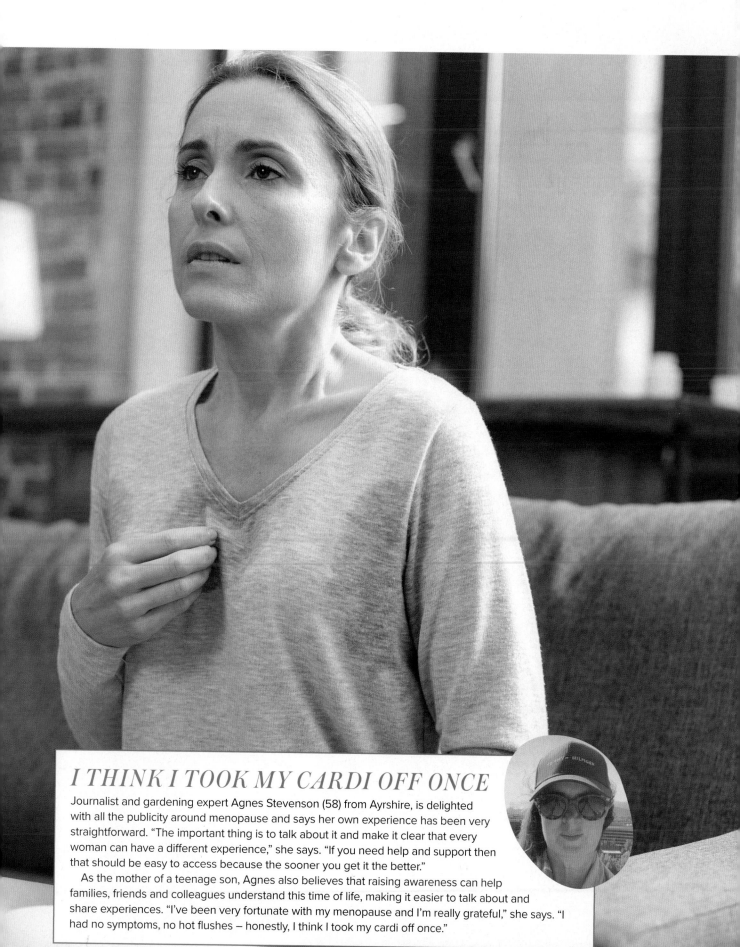

I THINK I TOOK MY CARDI OFF ONCE

Journalist and gardening expert Agnes Stevenson (58) from Ayrshire, is delighted with all the publicity around menopause and says her own experience has been very straightforward. "The important thing is to talk about it and make it clear that every woman can have a different experience," she says. "If you need help and support then that should be easy to access because the sooner you get it the better."

As the mother of a teenage son, Agnes also believes that raising awareness can help families, friends and colleagues understand this time of life, making it easier to talk about and share experiences. "I've been very fortunate with my menopause and I'm really grateful," she says. "I had no symptoms, no hot flushes – honestly, I think I took my cardi off once."

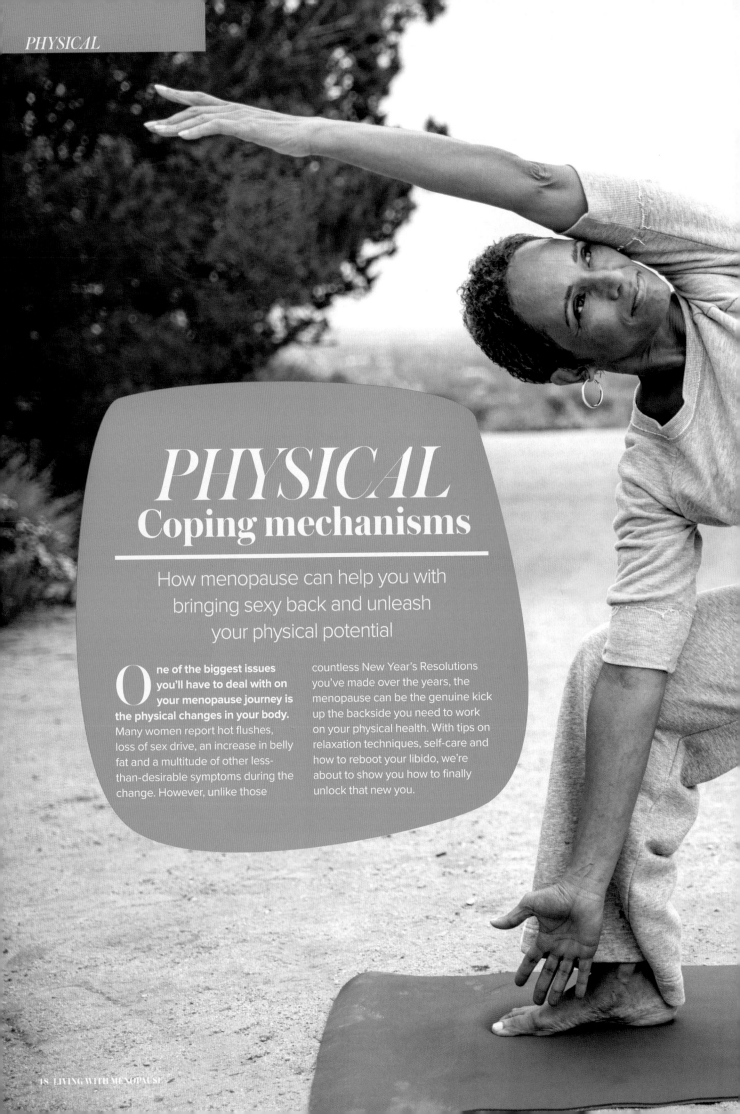

PHYSICAL
Coping mechanisms

How menopause can help you with
bringing sexy back and unleash
your physical potential

One of the biggest issues you'll have to deal with on your menopause journey is the physical changes in your body. Many women report hot flushes, loss of sex drive, an increase in belly fat and a multitude of other less-than-desirable symptoms during the change. However, unlike those countless New Year's Resolutions you've made over the years, the menopause can be the genuine kick up the backside you need to work on your physical health. With tips on relaxation techniques, self-care and how to reboot your libido, we're about to show you how to finally unlock that new you.

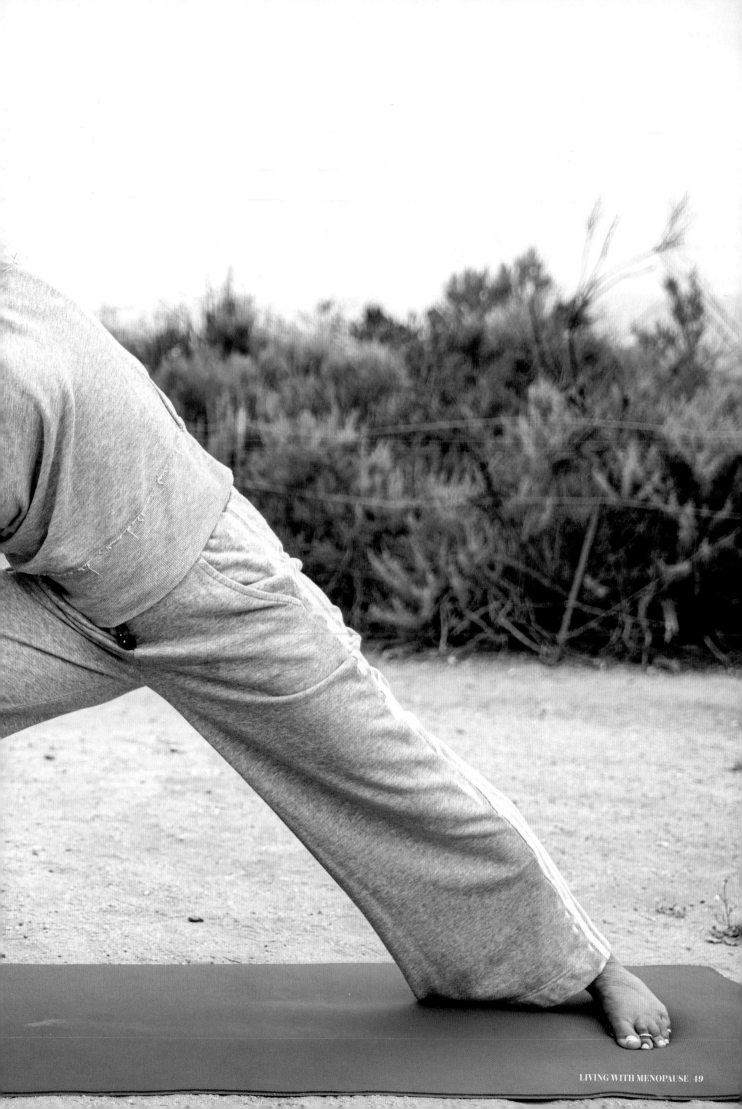

Fitness
THROUGH THE MENOPAUSE

An expert guide to the best workouts for women going through the change

Words by Fiona Russell

We're all aware that exercise is key to physical and mental well-being throughout our lives, but during the menopause it is even more critical for good health.

Declining hormones can cause a long list of symptoms, including weight gain (especially around the midriff), decreased muscle mass, reduced bone density leading to osteoporosis, joint pain, inflammation, pelvic floor weakness, fatigue, insomnia, anxiety and memory and concentration problems.

But there is some good news. By understanding the benefits of different types of exercise, women can discover many ways to lessen the unwanted symptoms of menopause. One of the most important areas to focus on is maintaining and building muscle mass through strength and resistance training.

While women naturally lose muscle mass as they age, during the menopause oestrogen deficiency causes an even greater reduction. Muscle is an important metabolic driver, helping maintain healthy weight, and it is also protects bones and joints.

Other forms of exercise that offer menopausal health advantages include cardio and high-impact workouts, as well as yoga. In addition, regular outdoor activity offers further health benefits of being in a natural environment.

We asked several fitness experts to recommend five of the best forms of exercise for during and after menopause.

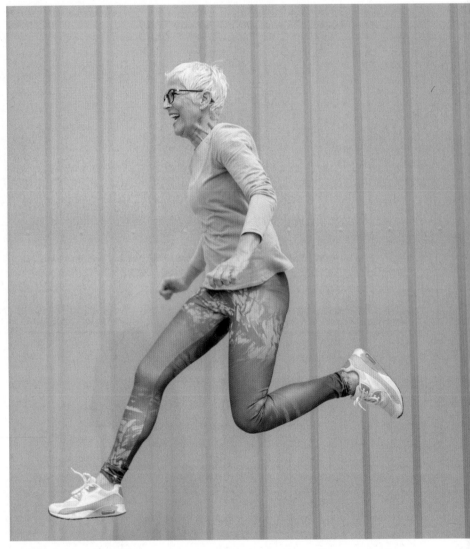

"By understanding the benefits of exercise, women can discover ways to lessen the unwanted symptoms of menopause"

CARDIO WORKOUTS

A drop in oestrogen levels can lead to a build-up of fat and cholesterol in the arteries, which can contribute to heart attacks and strokes. This means that cardio exercise – the type that makes your heart pump – is important.

Cardio workouts cover a wide range of activities, so you have plenty to choose from. They include: walking, jogging, running, hiking, cycling, swimming, dance and high-intensity gym-based sessions, such as HIIT (High-intensity interval training).

Lucy Gornall, a personal trainer with Healthspan Elite, is a big fan of walking, although she is clear: "it needs to be brisk walking".

She explains: "Walking is free and easy to do. It's great for getting your heart rate up and burning calories. Plus it releases the feel-good endorphins that clear your mind, it beats stress and anxiety and it can help to improve sleep."

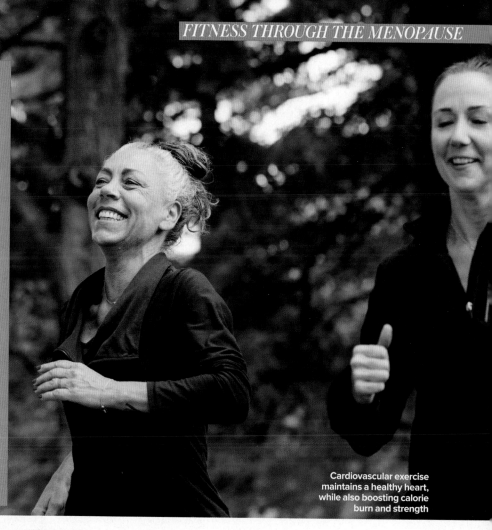

Cardiovascular exercise maintains a healthy heart, while also boosting calorie burn and strength

YOGA

A study at the University of California found that oestrogen directly affects the structure and function of muscles, ligaments and tendons. Therefore, when this hormone drops, the result is reduced flexibility and more aches and pains. That's why women complain of sore joints and muscles, slower recovery and feeling generally stiffer.

Piroska Cavell, who supports menopausal women with exercise and nutrition at well-being clinic Sese, recommends yoga for both physical and mental benefits. She says: "Yoga is fantastic for keeping your flexibility and also builds strength as you hold the poses. It is also great for calming the mind and improving your breathing."

Another study that considered the benefits of Hatha Yoga practice in menopause, uncovered its role in providing relief for some more specific symptoms, especially stress and depression.

Any kind of yoga will be beneficial to your health, but there are certain poses that are particularly suited for menopause. These include Shoulder Stand (Salamba Sarvangasana), Head-to-Knee Forward Bend (Janu Sirsasana), Reclining Bound Angle Pose (Supta Baddha Konasana), Downward-Facing Dog (Adho Mukha Svanasana), Reclining Hero Pose (Supta Virasana), and Bridge Pose (Setu Bandha Sarvangasana).

Try a non-impact exercise that focuses on flexibility and balance, in addition to strength

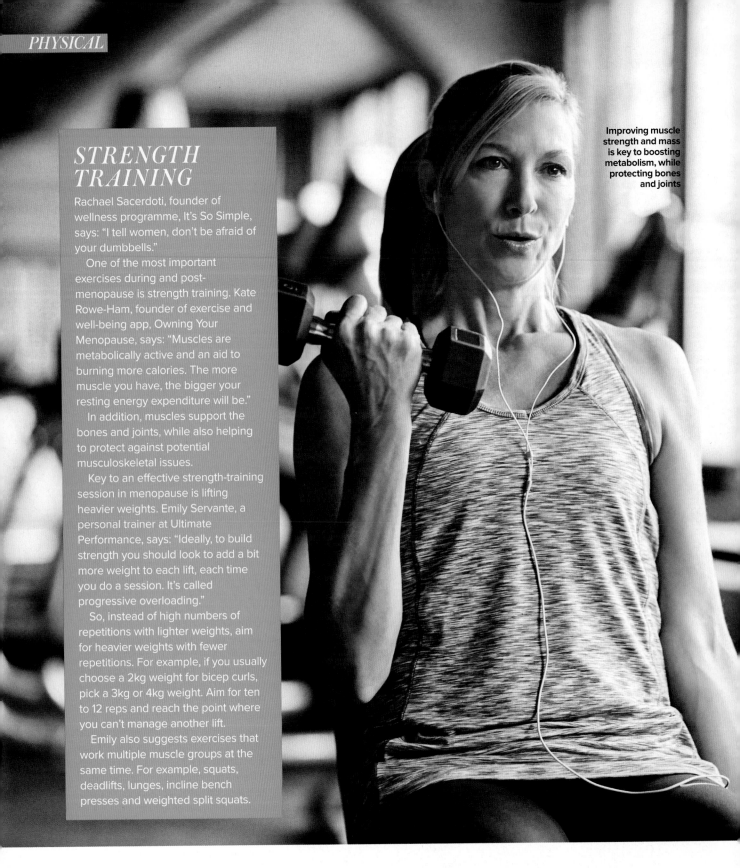

STRENGTH TRAINING

Rachael Sacerdoti, founder of wellness programme, It's So Simple, says: "I tell women, don't be afraid of your dumbbells."

One of the most important exercises during and post-menopause is strength training. Kate Rowe-Ham, founder of exercise and well-being app, Owning Your Menopause, says: "Muscles are metabolically active and an aid to burning more calories. The more muscle you have, the bigger your resting energy expenditure will be."

In addition, muscles support the bones and joints, while also helping to protect against potential musculoskeletal issues.

Key to an effective strength-training session in menopause is lifting heavier weights. Emily Servante, a personal trainer at Ultimate Performance, says: "Ideally, to build strength you should look to add a bit more weight to each lift, each time you do a session. It's called progressive overloading."

So, instead of high numbers of repetitions with lighter weights, aim for heavier weights with fewer repetitions. For example, if you usually choose a 2kg weight for bicep curls, pick a 3kg or 4kg weight. Aim for ten to 12 reps and reach the point where you can't manage another lift.

Emily also suggests exercises that work multiple muscle groups at the same time. For example, squats, deadlifts, lunges, incline bench presses and weighted split squats.

Improving muscle strength and mass is key to boosting metabolism, while protecting bones and joints

"*Muscles are metabolically active and an aid to burning more calories. The more muscle you have, the bigger your resting energy expenditure will be*"

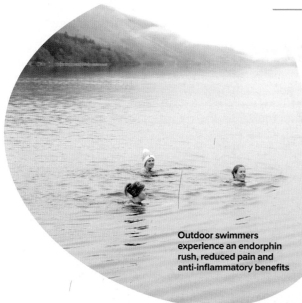

Outdoor swimmers experience an endorphin rush, reduced pain and anti-inflammatory benefits

OPEN WATER SWIMMING

Taking a dip in a lake, loch, river or the sea is increasingly popular – and swimmers talk of many health advantages including increased alertness and energy levels, plus the release of endorphins.

In addition, there are further claimed benefits, such as strengthening your immune system, an anti-inflammatory effect and increased blood flow. All of the above will be a real bonus during the menopause.

If you decide to give it a go, it is important to choose a safe place to swim and always go with at least one other person. Build up the time you spend in cold water, especially if you are planning to swim without a wetsuit.

Then, you can choose whether you will be a quick dipper or if you will aim for longer-distance swims. However, the more you go, the greater the benefits are said to be.

HIGH-IMPACT EXERCISE

Menopause significantly speeds up bone loss and increases the risk of osteoporosis. In fact, osteoporosis is said to be the primary disease in postmenopausal women.

The best way to preserve bone mass is to do high-impact exercises. The body stimulates bone growth through the process of the impact, such as when you are doing activities that cause you to change directions, make quick turns or jump.

Exercises include playing tennis, football or netball, trail running, hill and mountain hiking, some high-energy gym sessions and dances, as well as simple rope skipping.

Plyometrics, which is a type of exercise training that uses speed and force of different movements to build muscle power, is also good for bone density. Don't forget that vitamin D and calcium are crucial to bone health, too.

MY MENOPAUSE FITNESS

Outdoor journalist and blogger, Fiona Russell (www.fionaoutdoors.co.uk), found fitness helped her thrive during the menopause

When severe leg muscle cramps stopped me in my fitness tracks in my mid-40s, my mood plummeted. Through my own online research, I discovered that a drop in hormones associated with perimenopause might be to blame. I also realised I had many other menopause symptoms, including low mood, migraines, itchy skin, heavy periods, reduced libido, vaginal dryness, sweats and anxiety.

I was fortunate that HRT improved many of the issues but I'm also convinced that my passion for spending time outdoors, whether trail running, hiking, wild swimming, kayaking or skiing, have contributed to a happier decade.

Now 54, I feel fit (for my age!) and I am fairly happy with my weight. I add regular circuit training sessions to my regime in order to maintain my muscles and tone. I also have made new friends through my sports and enjoy the mental health benefits of spending a lot of time in a natural environment.

I am not going to tell all women to move to the Scottish Highlands in their menopause, but, for me, being close to an amazing outdoors playground has been key to my continued zest for life and happiness.

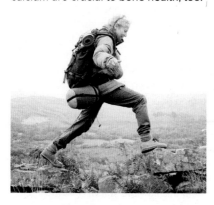

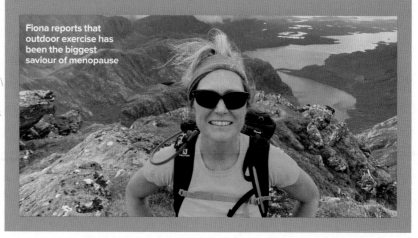

Fiona reports that outdoor exercise has been the biggest saviour of menopause

Alleviate symptoms with
YOGA

Yoga is a wonderful cure-all for a wide range of complaints and problems, and the symptoms of menopause are by no means any exception

Words by Natalie Denton

Yoga is for everyone. From complete beginners to seasoned yogis, the zenful discipline is designed to allow you to listen to what your body can do, and help you build on that, little by little. Yoga is all positive. There are no drawbacks – only a wealth of health benefits for the body and mind. For instance, stretching is incredible for increasing flexibility and gently loosening any muscle aches and pains that menopause brings your way. Holding poses can feel like a workout, but over time they will help to boost muscle strength, enhance bone density and improve circulation. Not only will this make you feel fitter and stronger, but it can help with problems that arise from declining levels of oestrogen, such as the increased risks of cardiovascular disease, osteoporosis and weight gain. Also, the flood of endorphins that comes not only from exercise, but yoga's focus on deep breathing and meditation, can bolster your mood (helping to alleviate 'menorage'), alleviate hot flushes, relieve stress and even improve sleep.

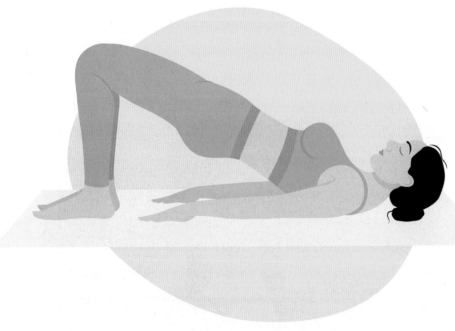

BRIDGE POSE

Bridge Pose is a wonderful muscle-building stretch that improves posture, especially perfect for those who sit for long periods of the day, or who suffer from lower back pain. While it helps to strengthen the back, bottom, and legs, Bridge Pose is also great for the pelvis, and offers you an opportunity to squeeze in (excuse the pun) a few pelvic floor exercises. Both techniques help to combat incontinence issues menopause may have brought your way. Begin lying on your back with your arms at your side, palms face down. Bend your knees, bringing your feet as close to your bottom as possible, then lift your hips. To increase the benefit of this pose, place a block, cushion, or towel between your knees and keep firmly in place. Hold the pose for ten seconds then lower, gently curling through the spine.

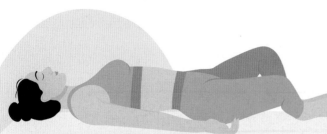

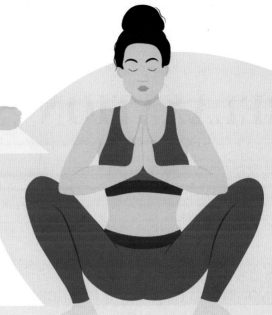

RECLINING BOUND ANGLE POSE
(SUPTA BADDHA KONASANA)

Also known as the Butterfly Pose, the Reclining Bound Angle Pose is super for opening up your entire torso, allowing the chest, lungs, heart, abdomen and pelvis to benefit from this beautiful stretch, which as a byproduct helps to lower the feelings of stress and improves mood. If you're new to yoga, try this pose seated, with your heels pressed together and your knees open to the sides, as close to the floor as you feel comfortable. When this position is no longer a challenge, recline so that you're laying back to elongate the stretch, with your palms facing the ceiling. You may feel more comfortable using pillows to support your head and knees to begin with.

MALASANA

Also referred to as the Hindu Squat, Malasana is a particularly wonderful pose if menopause has lowered your libido or caused vaginal dryness, because it stretches the thighs, groin and hips, plus tones the core and increases circulation to the pelvis, helping to stimulate sexual energy. Stand with your feet a touch wider than your hips and point your feet out 45 degrees. Lower all the way down into a squat position, keeping your knees in line with your toes until your bottom is just inches away from the floor. Press your palms together and elbows into the sides of your knees. With your breath, push your knees wider apart. With time you may like to progress this stretch by lifting your heels off the floor.

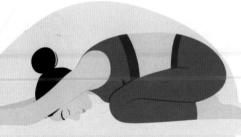

CHILD'S POSE

There's no other stretch quite like the beautiful Child's Pose for causing a warming swell of endorphins to flood your body as it stretches and relaxes, perfect for when you're feeling overwhelmed, lethargic or stressed. As well as calming the mind, it's superb for stretching out the spine and hips. Simply begin sitting on your knees, then open them out to the sides and lean your torso forward towards the ground with your arms stretching out in front of you. It may take time for you to reach the ground with your torso comfortably, so start out with a pillow underneath you. Hold for as long as feels comfortable or is needed.

SAVASANA

To the untrained eye, Savasana may just look like someone is having a lie down, but there's more to it. Savasana is perfect for letting go, clearing your mind and just being in the moment. Mindfulness is crucial for combating the mental toll menopause can wreak on your mood and mind and this pose is your ticket out of the darkness. Lay on your back, legs and arms straight with your feet a little wider than your hips and your palms facing the ceiling. Breathe in through your nose for three seconds, allowing your belly to rise. Hold it a beat. Then gently exhale for five seconds, actively deflating your stomach towards the spine. After a few repetitions, try exhaling with a slow "haaa" sound. Aim to keep your mind clear of thoughts by only focusing on your breathing.

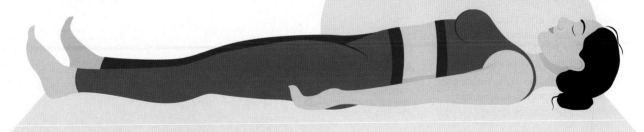

RELAXATION
Techniques

Some simple-but-powerful methods to try when
you need to grasp a moment of calm

Words by Ella Carter

DEEP BREATHING

It may sound simple, but taking a moment to do some deep breathing can make a huge difference to reducing symptoms like night sweats, insomnia and anxiety. This is because it delivers more oxygen to our brains and slows the heart rate. Try the 4-7-8 method for reducing stress: fully exhale, then breathe in through your nose for the count of four, hold it for a count of seven, then exhale through your mouth for a count of eight. Repeat three or four times.

PROGRESSIVE MUSCLE RELAXATION

This technique is ideal for when you can't sleep, or for when you feel tightly wound or anxious. Lie on your back somewhere comfortable, and bring your attention to your body. Start at your toes – tense all the muscles and then release and relax. Then tense the rest of your muscles in your feet, and relax. Gradually repeat the process, working your way up your body from your toes to your face. If you have any pain or injuries, just skip these areas to be safe.

MINDFULNESS AND MEDITATION

Mindfulness is all about focusing on the sensation and feeling that your body is experiencing in the moment, and not letting your mind skip about, worrying about things in the future or the past. This is tricky to master, but trying meditation can be a great way to

start. There are plenty of apps out there to help you, but the name of the game is to focus on your breathing and to be kind to your mind. If it starts to wander, lead it back to your breath.

YOGA

Gentle stretching – even just ten minutes a day – can help with both physical and psychological symptoms of menopause. Yoga is a great way to take some time for yourself and to let any tension or stress that you're holding on to melt away. It's also a good low-impact exercise, which is important for overall health and wellbeing. If you're already a yogi, embrace your mat! Or if you're a beginner, join a class or look for an instructional video to be guided through the basics.

PACED RESPIRATION

This breathing technique can help with hot flushes. It's about lowering your breathing rate to around six to eight breaths per minute – which takes a

little practice when we usually take around 15 breaths in that time. Begin by breathing in for a slow count of five, then breathing out for the same count. Try to do this morning and evening to practise, and then when you feel any vasomotor symptoms coming on (like night sweats or hot flushes), employ this method to ease your stress and see you through.

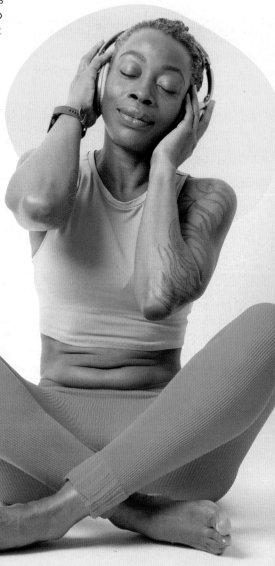

Life can be overwhelming. Finding ways to relax and breathe is important when it all feels a bit much

PRESS PAUSE
(on your menopause)

Escape for a few days and
emerge feeling like yourself again
with a menopause retreat

Words by Rebecca Bradbury

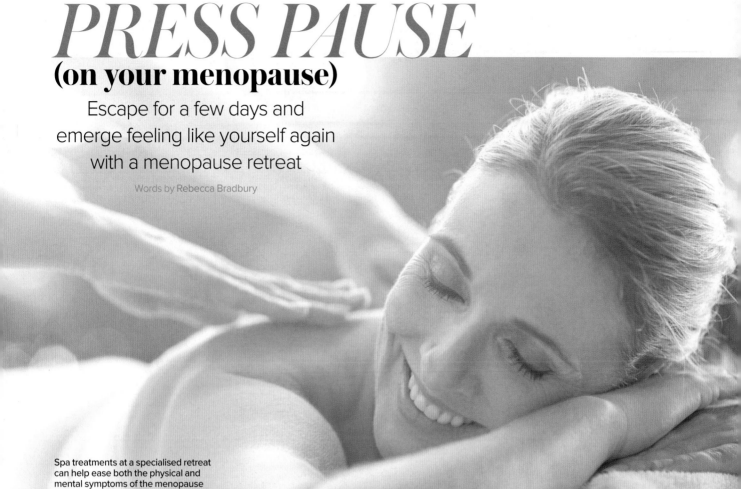

Spa treatments at a specialised retreat
can help ease both the physical and
mental symptoms of the menopause

The stresses and strains of the menopause can sometimes become too much to bear. Not only do a whole host of bodily changes begin to take their toll over time, but the emotional symptoms can have an overwhelming effect too. Never is a relaxing getaway needed more than during this transition, and thankfully menopause retreats can cater to this demand.

Often set in sumptuous surroundings, these women-focused getaways offer a complete escape from the outside world. Settings can range from beachside havens, to luxurious five-star spas, to countryside mansions. But all aim to provide a holistic way of embracing the changes and navigating the difficulties associated with this time of life.

With such dreamy grounds, these retreats are also perfect for exploring by foot, allowing guests to combine walking with immersion in nature, both of which have many positive benefits on physical health and mental wellbeing. Similarly, yoga, Pilates and other exercise sessions specifically suited to menopausal women are often part of the programme.

Another major draw of these getaways are spa treatments aimed at those in their 40s and 50s, with massages and facials among some of the popular treatments available, along with saunas reported to help manage hot flushes.

Experts are regularly on hand, too, sharing the tools needed to adapt to the menopause. Hypnotherapists, nutritionists and personal trainers are just a few examples of the professionals usually found at menopausal retreats around the world, with many offering bespoke therapy, personal eating plans and tailored fitness programmes.

Meditation and mindfulness sessions are also regular fixtures on the agenda, with an emphasis on relaxation, de-stressing and improving mental health to be expected.

Whether women stay for one night or one week, they are guaranteed to leave refreshed, revitalised and ready to embrace the changes coming up in the next stage of their life.

TOP OF THE RETREATS

One leading wellness hotel specialising in menopause retreats is Preidlhof in northern Italy

Ancient healing sessions, sumptuous spa treatments and invigorating yoga are just some of the activities on offer at this idyllic wellness hotel. Helping guests find balance and reconnect with themselves, this is an ultimate wellness destination for those needing a break from the menopause. *tinyurl.com/3krxpjcb*

Image credit: Laura La Monaca

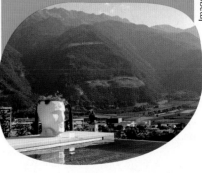

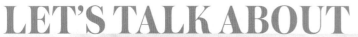

LET'S TALK ABOUT

Sex!

Despite what you might hear, the menopause doesn't mean the end of your love life

Words by Sophie Barton

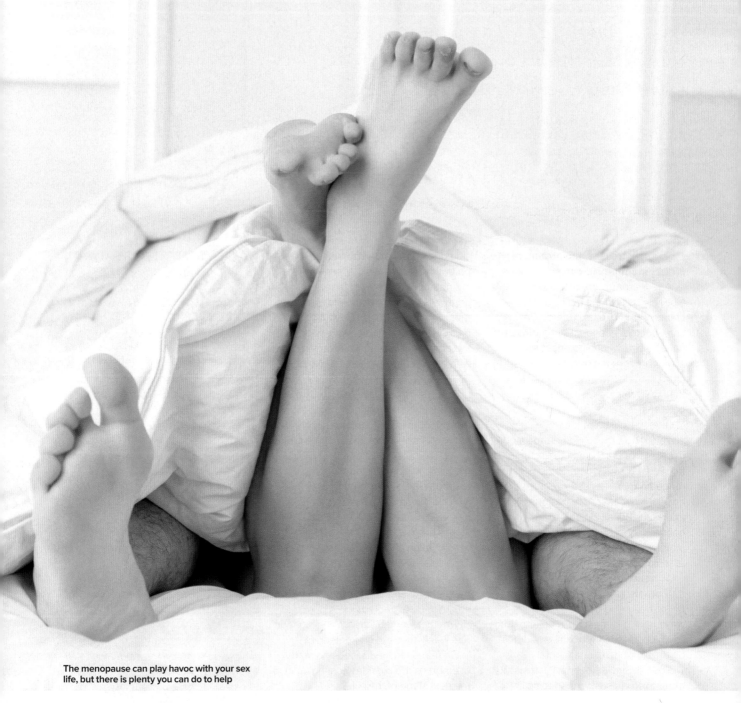

The menopause can play havoc with your sex life, but there is plenty you can do to help

We often link the menopause to hot flushes, brain fog and low mood, but many women find it impacts their love life too. Let's face it, it's hard to feel up for it when you're struggling with night sweats, sleeping badly and feeling anxious – then there's vaginal dryness to contend with as well.

But whether you're struggling with a lack of libido or sexual discomfort, rest assured that these are perfectly normal – if undesirable – side effects. In fact, one study found that 42 percent of women transitioning into menopause reported symptoms of sexual dysfunction, while after eight years, the number rose to 88 percent.

"Testosterone levels naturally decline throughout a woman's lifetime, and oestrogen levels tend to drop sharply around the time of the menopause, both of which can affect your libido," explains Dr Bryony Henderson, lead GP at digital healthcare provider, Livi (**livi.co.uk**).

"Falling oestrogen also reduces the natural vaginal secretions that a woman produces, leading to dry vaginal tissue that can be uncomfortable and even painful during sex. Vaginal dryness – also called vaginal atrophy, affects more than 50 percent of postmenopausal women, and can cause stinging and itchiness too. Meanwhile, dropping progesterone levels can lead to sleep issues, irritability and anxiety."

This might paint a grim picture, but it's not all doom and gloom. While the menopause may change the way you experience sex, there's plenty you can do to create a healthy love life that works for you. Here's how...

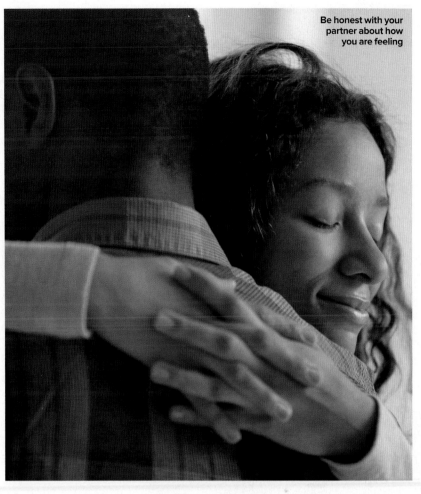

Be honest with your partner about how you are feeling

LUBRICATE

If intercourse feels uncomfortable, don't panic. "During menopause, dropping oestrogen levels mean less lubrication (and less blood flow) to your vagina, which can lead to painful sex or difficulty when trying to get aroused," explains Pippa Murphy, sex and relationship expert

at condoms.uk. "Fortunately though, there are ways to combat the effects of vaginal dryness, and the quickest is to use a lubricant." You'll find plenty of options available over the counter and online, many of which will do a great job of boosting arousal and helping to decrease discomfort.

TRY VAGINAL OESTROGEN

Dr Henderson recommends making an appointment with your doctor, to find a prescription treatment that works for you. She explains, "Vaginal oestrogen, which is available as a cream, ring or pessary, can be placed inside your vagina to relieve dryness." These treatments can safely be used alongside HRT. "Some studies also show that women who take HRT report higher sexual desire," adds Dr Henderson.

TALK ABOUT IT

It may not be your favourite topic of conversation, but if your partner isn't clued up about the menopause, they won't understand how you're feeling. Pippa says, "Try explaining more about what happens physiologically during this time in a woman's life: hot flushes, mood swings, vaginal dryness etc. Plus, it doesn't matter how long your relationship has been going on or how well you think you know each other's bodies, people's desires change over time. So, speak to your partner about how you're feeling and how they can better cater to your needs. If your self-esteem has taken a dip because of a change in your appearance, ask your partner what they find sexy about you, and return the compliment. This will give you both a confidence boost."

BUILD INTIMACY

If penetrative sex hurts, it can put you off intimacy altogether. If this is the case, Pippa suggests focusing on smaller acts of intimacy, such as holding hands,

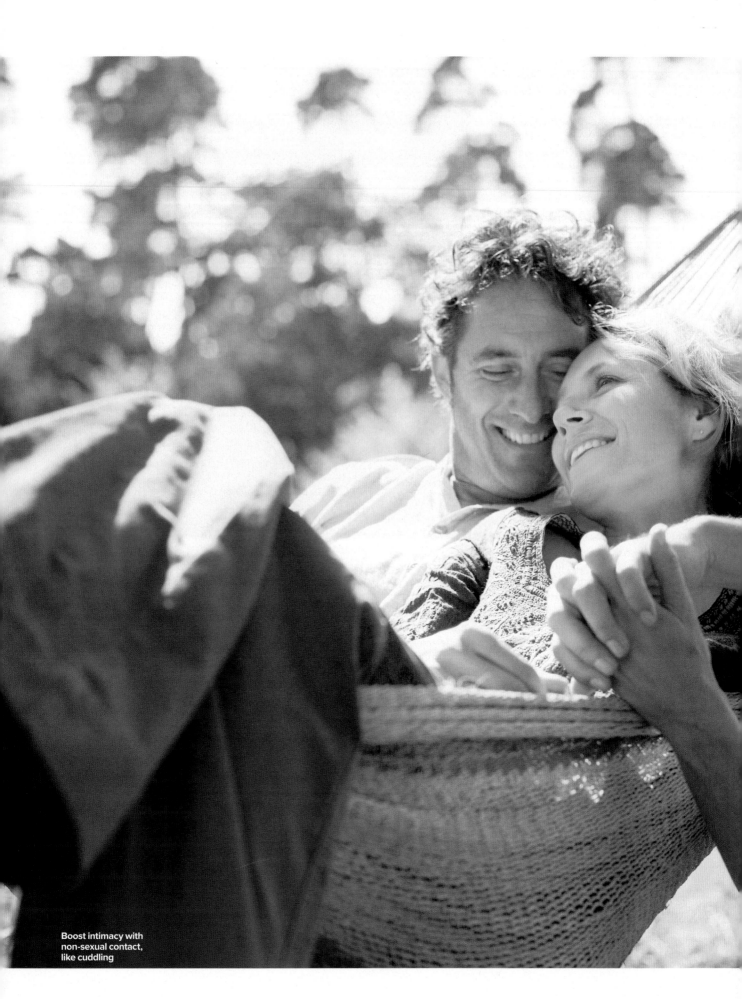

Boost intimacy with
non-sexual contact,
like cuddling

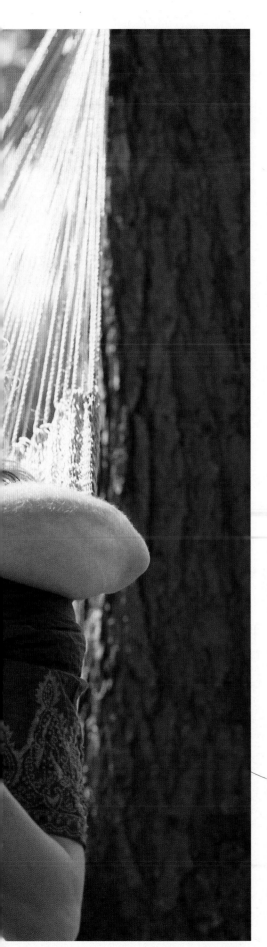

"Sex toys, especially vibrators, promote blood flow to your vagina"

kissing, hugging or even massaging. She explains, "All of these smaller acts of touch help release oxytocin, otherwise known as the bonding hormone, which puts you more at ease.

"And if you're not feeling up for sex, don't fret. There's a common misconception that sex is intimacy, but that couldn't be further from the truth. Instead, focus on building non-sexual intimacy by making time for a date day or night every single week. If you're fatigued, this could be something as simple as cooking a nice meal together. These intimate memories will help build a stronger bond."

CHECK OUT TOYS

Sex toys might sound scary, but they're actually a fantastic way to increase arousal and also show your partner what you like. Barbara Santini, psychologist and sex advisor at **peachesandscreams.co.uk** says, "Sex toys, especially vibrators, promote blood flow to your vagina. When you are sensitive down there, you are more likely to enjoy sex. Take your time to find what works for you best – you can achieve that through masturbation."

MANAGE STRESS

If you find yourself stressed or anxious during the menopause, this can dampen feelings of sexual desire – it's hard for your brain to process both

feelings at once. It's important to take action to manage your stress levels, such as breathing exercises, taking time out to relax with friends and going for regular walks outdoors. Pippa adds, "Studies have shown that 20 to 30 minutes of physical activity can not only enhance your emotional health but your sex drive, too. This is because exercise gets your blood moving and releases endorphins, which trigger a positive feeling in your body.

SWITCH POSITION

Pippa recommends trying out different positions, until you find something that feels good for both of you. "As sex during menopause can be painful, you may not want the deepest thrusts," she says.

"Getting on top allows you to control the depth and pace of penetration – it allows you to decide. Try leaning over a counter or table and asking your partner to enter you from behind, too. This position allows you to control the depth of penetration, plus your partner has easy access to your erogenous zones, such as your nipples, neck or back, which can then turn you on more."

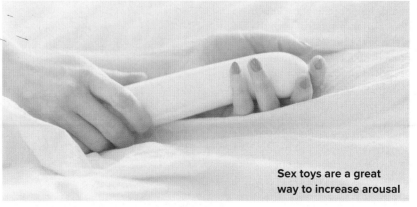

Sex toys are a great way to increase arousal

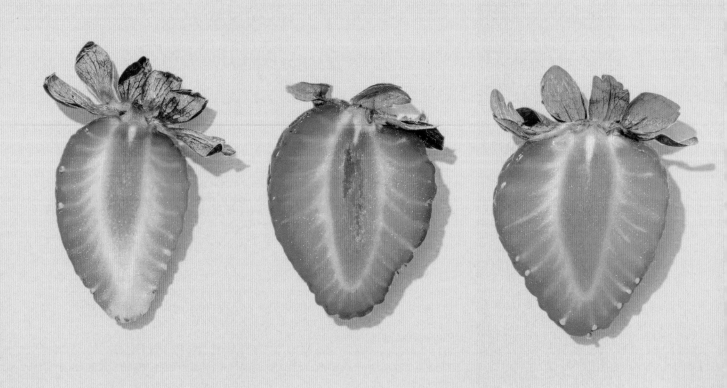

WHAT'S UP
down there?

Fluctuating hormones during menopause can cause changes to your vagina, vulva and bladder – here's what's going on and why

Words by Ella Carter

The range of symptoms that can affect your nether regions during menopause and perimenopause are known as genitourinary syndrome of the menopause, or GSM. They're all brought about by the drop in oestrogen produced by your ovaries.

GSM is more common than you might think, but can often go misdiagnosed or unreported. No matter what you're feeling, don't be embarrassed – have a chat with your doctor about any of these symptoms for help and advice.

A CHANGE IN SIZE OR SHAPE

Don't worry – this doesn't happen overnight, but it is something that can change over time. Oestrogen is responsible for keeping the tissues that make up your vagina elastic and supple. Once these hormone levels drop, this means that the skin around your vagina might get thinner, drier and more delicate. Blood flow is also reduced to the area, and this combination of factors can cause your vagina to reduce in size. You might notice a change in your vulva, as fat deposits may reduce. Plus you might notice pubic hair getting thinner.

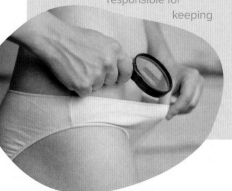

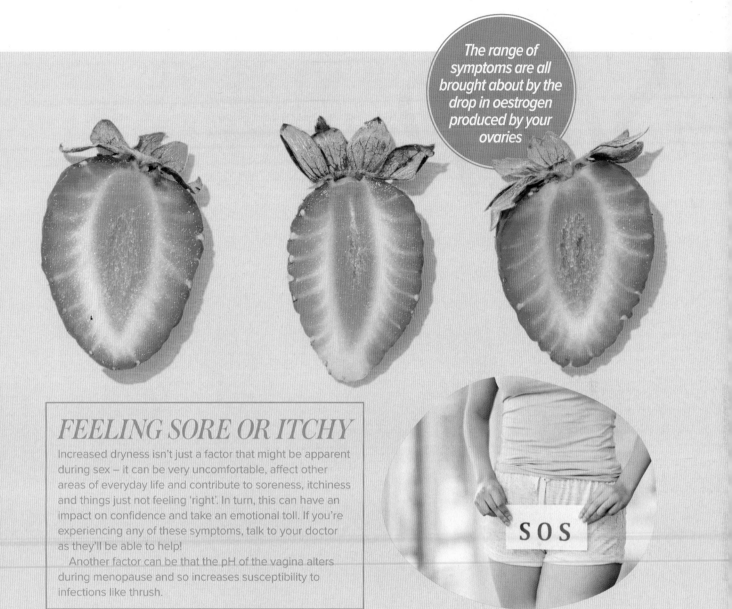

The range of symptoms are all brought about by the drop in oestrogen produced by your ovaries

FEELING SORE OR ITCHY

Increased dryness isn't just a factor that might be apparent during sex – it can be very uncomfortable, affect other areas of everyday life and contribute to soreness, itchiness and things just not feeling 'right'. In turn, this can have an impact on confidence and take an emotional toll. If you're experiencing any of these symptoms, talk to your doctor as they'll be able to help!

Another factor can be that the pH of the vagina alters during menopause and so increases susceptibility to infections like thrush.

SOS

DRYNESS

Oestrogen levels are also responsible for lubrication, which is produced by glands near the cervix and at the entrance to the vagina. The reduction in hormones means that these glands are less active and reduce in number during and after menopause, which causes dryness.

INCONTINENCE

Dropping levels of oestrogen can weaken muscles, which affects the pelvic floor – the group of muscles that support your organs down there. The bladder can get squashed, so you might need to pee more, with more urgency. The bladder valve can also be affected, which means there can be a leak when you laugh or exercise.

URINARY TRACT INFECTIONS

Before menopause, oestrogen stimulates cells that line the vagina to produce glycogen – a substance that helps maintain good bacteria that can fight infection. Once glycogen levels drop, coupled with thinner vaginal tissues, the change in bacteria levels can make you more susceptible to infection, especially in the urinary tract. Be sure to keep drinking plenty of water, which will always help, and contact your doctor if you're experiencing regular UTIs.

PAIN DURING SEX

After menopause, the folds within the vagina that usually allow for expansion for childbirth and penetration, known as vaginal rugae, get thinner and flatter. This makes it much more delicate and, combined with increased dryness, can mean sex can hurt.

However, cutting out sex altogether can actually make this worse. Regular sex throughout menopause helps keep vaginal tissues strong and moist and means that your vagina can maintain its length and width.

Sleep AND THE MENOPAUSE

Insomnia, night sweats and how the menopause can greatly affect your sleep

Words by **Bee Ginger**

Sleep during the menopause is a vicious cycle; changes in hormone levels often cause disturbed sleep, and disturbed sleep can in turn alter hormone levels

SLEEP ISSUES THAT ARE COMMONLY ASSOCIATED WITH THE MENOPAUSE

Your menopause is a time of physical, hormonal and psychological change and can often greatly affect your sleep pattern. Not enough sleep can have a detrimental effect on cognitive functions, heart health, mental health, and even lead to osteoporosis. Recent studies have found that almost two-thirds of women going through the menopause suffer disrupted sleep and that most wake up approximately three times a night from heart palpitations, sweats, insomnia and restless leg syndrome. This can really add up over a period of time, with some studies suggesting that the average woman could lose as much as five-and-a-half weeks of sleep a year dependent on the length of her nightly menopause struggles. The majority of women were found to suffer from temperature issues (82 percent) while insomnia came in at 41 percent and heart palpitations 23 percent. As women progress into the late 40s and early 50s, an average of 40 percent will experience sleep issues. These issues become more common between perimenopause and postmenopause, with the most commonly reported sleep problems including insomnia, sleep-disordered breathing, mood changes and our old friend the hot flush. Here we take a look at the reasons behind these problems and offer some resolutions for getting the very best night's sleep possible.

HOT FLUSHES

Hot flushes can occur at any time and can last as long as five minutes. Those that occur at night are sometimes referred to as night sweats, and they are common with over 85 percent of women going through the menopause. This heating sensation causes the sufferer to wake up because of the rise in body temperature and increase in blood flow prior to a flush. Due to the increase in adrenaline and heat, you can feel greatly energised, which then makes it incredibly difficult to go back to sleep. Even if you are able to go back to sleep your quality of sleep suffers, often due to the discomfort of the flush and being woken up frequently during the night. The knock-on effect of this can be exhaustion the following day. Many women suffering extreme hot flushes have also reported having chronic insomnia. Hot flushes cause an increase in the heart rate and temperature of the skin. As the body tries to reduce its temperature you begin to perspire. You may also experience dizziness and heart palpitations during a flush.

INSOMNIA

As we age our sleep cycle begins to change. It is no longer as consistent as it was in our youth, when we could sleep anywhere and at any time of the day. We now begin to tire earlier and in turn wake up much earlier than before, which means less hours of deep and restorative sleep. It also explains why more women, particularly those embarking on the menopause, suffer from insomnia. Anyone experiencing sleep deprivation or insomnia knows that it is no joke. All those hours tossing and turning and staring at the ceiling, only to fall asleep minutes before the alarm clock goes off is soul destroying. The day that follows is a mixture of fatigue, anxiety and feelings of irritability, and it's often the cause of headaches. Although insomnia is common in both sexes, the number of sufferers increases greatly with women entering the menopause.

MENOPAUSE AND YOUR SLEEP HORMONES

When a woman's ovaries cease to produce oestrogen and progesterone, the menopause really steps up a gear, as those are the hormones that affect so many things in our bodies, from digestion to mood and most

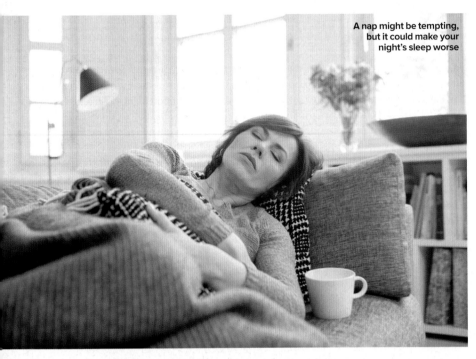

A nap might be tempting, but it could make your night's sleep worse

"Sleep apnea and snoring occur most commonly in postmenopausal women"

importantly sleep! Oestrogen plays an integral role; not only does it regulate our temperature to keep our body cool at night but it also helps to metabolise serotonin (the chemical that transports messages between the nerve cells in our brain throughout the body, among other things) and can even act as an antidepressant. Therefore less oestrogen results in a poorer mood and higher temperatures, leading to a lower quality of sleep. The decline of oestrogen in our bodies contributes greatly to our disrupted sleep, causing night sweats, hot flushes, depressed mood, anxiety and waking up early in the morning. Aches and pains in our joints and bladder problems at night are also a common cause of oestrogen decline, which then interrupt our ability to sleep. Less progesterone also plays a part in causing sleep disturbance, as it has a sleep-inducing effect on our body, and a decline in progesterone impacts the secretion of melatonin, which can compound sleep issues.

MELATONIN: YOUR BODY'S NATURAL SLEEP HORMONE

Melatonin is most commonly thought of as a sleep supplement. It can, however, treat other symptoms of your menopause. Contrary to common belief, it is not in fact a sedative but a hormone that can help the body to better regulate its sleep cycles and biological clock. It is naturally produced in our bodies; however as we reach perimenopause our body begins to produce less of it. The same thing happens with oestrogen, progesterone and cortisol (the fight or flight hormone that elevates during the night, causing added stress and worry). One solution

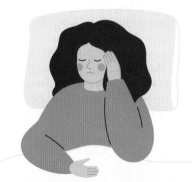

is to take a supplement to aid the sleep process. By creating a regular sleep schedule, melatonin can shorten the time it takes for you to drift off – so no more counting sheep! It has also been proven to help reduce fatigue and sleepiness during the day. Melatonin boasts strong antioxidant powers, helping to protect against cell damage in the brain and body. Research has found that it can even be used to help prevent and delay memory loss and cognitive impairment, which are other issues experienced while journeying through the menopause.

SLEEP APNOEA AND RESTLESS LEG SYNDROME

Research has found that due to a decline in progesterone in postmenopausal women, many begin to suffer with sleep apnoea and snoring. This can also lead to other hormonal changes that can prevent the muscles in the upper airways from relaxing, therefore obstructing breathing and causing lapses in sleep. This then results in low mood, headaches, irritability and even more tiredness.

Sleep apnea and snoring occur most commonly in postmenopausal women. Another condition linked to the menopause is restless leg syndrome. This is where you feel a constant tingling in your legs, making you keep wanting to move them. Due to these sensations and involuntary movements, the sufferer keeps waking up, making it hard to fall back asleep.

BREAK THE CYCLE

Sleep and mood disorders are like being trapped in a vicious cycle. If you already suffer from stress, anxiety or depression then you are more likely to suffer from insomnia. Those already suffering from insomnia are more at risk of anxiety and depression due to their lack of sleep. The ongoing pattern can be hard to break, especially as the effects continue throughout the day. Cognitive behavioural therapy (CBT) can be effective in relieving these symptoms of menopause. By working with a trained therapist, you'll learn to recognise behaviours and thoughts that are impacting your sleep and unlearn any unhealthy behaviours, thereby helping you to improve your sleep.

HANDY TIPS FOR
BETTER SLEEP

- ◆ Start by following a regular sleep schedule. Try going to bed at the same time every night and getting up at the same time each morning. Try not to take any naps, as these could interfere with you being able to sleep at night.

- ◆ It might sound obvious, but make sure to visit the toilet before going to bed to try and avoid having to get up during the night, which inevitably wakes you up fully. Also try to avoid drinking anything a few hours before you hit the hay.

- ◆ Try to follow a healthy diet and maintain a steady weight. A lot of women do gain weight after the menopause and higher weights can cause obstructive sleep apnea (OSA). Stay clear of acidic and spicy foods, as they can trigger hot flushes.

- ◆ Create a cool bedroom environment by placing a fan next to your bed or leaving the window open to circulate fresh air.

- ◆ Give alcohol, nicotine and caffeine a miss, especially in the evening, as they are known to impede falling – and staying – asleep.

- ◆ Develop a nighttime routine for falling back asleep following a night sweat. Keep a change of clothes nearby and a glass of water at hand and try not to get up or switch on the lights.

- ◆ Take a bath, read or listen to music to help you destress before bed. Meditation and deep breathing are both good relaxation techniques.

- ◆ Sleep naked or wear cool fabrics made from natural materials like cotton. Choose the same fabric for your bed sheets.

- ◆ Stress and anxious thoughts can keep your mind whirling at night, making sleep impossible. Exercise and yoga can help, or talk to a health professional for some advice on lifestyle changes and stress relief.

With a bit of planning, you could sleep once more!

CLOSE TO THE
BONE

Menopause is a critical time for a woman's
bone health, as this article reveals

Words by Rebecca Bradbury

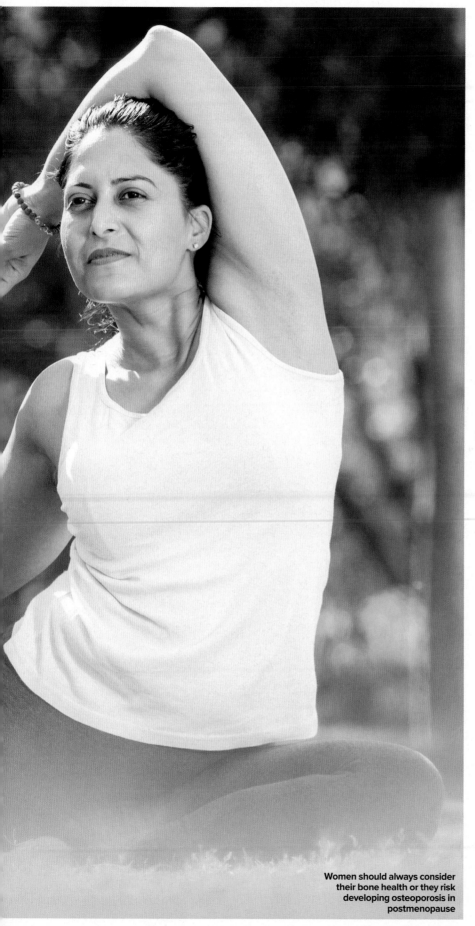

Women should always consider their bone health or they risk developing osteoporosis in postmenopause

"It's estimated women lose up to 10% of their bone mass in the first five years after menopause"

Some symptoms of the menopause are impossible to ignore. For example, night sweats, hot flushes and mood changes are infamous for their overwhelming intensity. Yet other side effects go unnoticed for years, despite causing longer-term health issues for women.

Among these 'silent but deadly' symptoms is the loss of bone mass, which is problematic because it puts postmenopausal women at a higher risk of developing osteoporosis.

The menopause also causes joint stiffness and pain for some, while a loss of muscle mass and strength happens naturally as we age. Mix all of these changes together and it's easy to understand exactly why bone health needs to be made a priority for women, especially as they approach middle age.

Exploring how fluctuating levels of oestrogen can affect the skeletal system, in addition to how the associated aches and pains can be managed and prevented, will give women the confidence they need to cope at this time.

MENOPAUSE AND OSTEOPOROSIS

Women reach peak bone mass between the ages of 25 and 30, when the skeleton has stopped growing. Bones are at their strongest and thickest at this time, but after the age of 30, the body can't replace bone cells as quickly as they're lost – a process unfortunately accelerated by the menopause.

Declining oestrogen levels are to blame for this loss of bone mass, (surprise surprise!) as the hormone helps slow down the natural breakdown of bone. Less oestrogen means it cannot perform its inhibitive effect as effectively and, as a result, bone density begins to decrease.

This puts postmenopausal women at a higher risk of developing osteoporosis, a condition where bones weaken, making them fragile and more likely to break. Research suggests that one in two women over the age of 60 will experience at least one fracture due to osteoporosis. Not only are these injuries painful, but they are also associated with a decreased quality of life and increased mortality.

As bone loss occurs without any symptoms, osteoporosis is usually only detected when a sudden bump or fall causes a fracture. With the diagnosis happening at this late stage, women need to start taking their bone health seriously as early as possible.

IMPROVING BONE STRENGTH

Thankfully, there are a number of lifestyle changes women can make to lower their chances of developing osteoporosis. Regular exercise, particularly weight-bearing activities such as walking, running, tennis or weight-training, is recommended for maintaining bone strength and mass.

A number of key nutrients are also essential for healthy bones. Top of the list is calcium, with the richest sources available in milk, cheese and yoghurt. But the mineral can only be effective if it is absorbed efficiently from food, which is

where vitamin D comes in – found in foods such as eggs, oily fish and certain fortified foods like breakfast cereals and plant-based drinks.

Protein and other nutrients including magnesium, vitamin K, phosphorus and potassium also have important parts to play in maintaining and increasing bone strength.

WOMEN AT HIGHER RISK

Sufficient calories are also needed or bones won't be able to get all their required nutrients. Therefore, malnutrition and being underweight may increase the risk of osteoporosis. Similarly, smoking, an excessive

> *"Women need to start taking their bone health seriously as early as possible"*

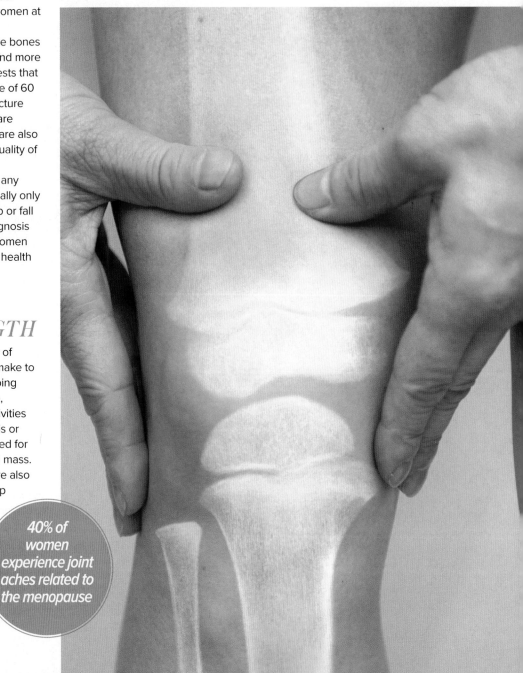

40% of women experience joint aches related to the menopause

alcohol intake and too much caffeine can also have an adverse impact on a person's bone health.

Those who experience an early menopause – before 45 years old and especially before 40 – are also at a higher risk of developing osteoporosis. For these women, the natural process of losing bone mass will be in motion for a much longer period of time.

JOINT PAIN

Bones are not the only part of the skeletal system that oestrogen affects. The hormone also helps take care of connective tissue, such as cartilage, and ensures joints are kept well lubricated. This explains why women with declining oestrogen levels will start experiencing pain and stiffness in their fingers, elbows and other joints. These could be new aches, but old injuries can flare up too.

Exacerbating the situation further is the fact that oestrogen also acts as an anti-inflammatory. Therefore, with less of the hormone in the body, the inflammation that occurs when cartilage in a joint naturally breaks down cannot be reduced as efficiently.

Unfortunately, these issues put women at risk of developing menopause-related osteoarthritis. Another blow is that the connection between the menopause and osteoarthritis is not fully understood, which makes it harder for the condition to be treated.

PREVENTION AND COPING STRATEGIES

Although more research is needed, maintaining a healthy weight, quitting smoking and eating foods rich in omega-3 or vitamins C and E are thought to help prevent menopause-related joint pain.

Movement is also key, although this might sound counterintuitive for women suffering from joint pain. Yet the menopause slows down the metabolism, which leads to weight gain, and being overweight makes arthritis even more difficult to manage.

Moderate to light activities, such as yoga, swimming and walking, are recommended, while simple at-home routines can help reduce menopausal joint pain. Treatments include gentle stretching, using ice packs or hot water bottles on sore areas, having a bath, and practising relaxation techniques and mindfulness. Over the counter medications, like painkillers and anti-inflammatory gels, can help too.

The importance of bone health for children and adolescents is widely acknowledged. Yet when it comes to the same topic for menopausal women, discussion is scarce, despite it being a vital concern.

Understanding why bone health should be a priority empowers women at any age to better protect themselves against menopause-related skeletal problems, such as osteoporosis and osteoarthritis. The good news is it's never too late to make the dietary and lifestyle changes required to improve bone and joint health.

OTHER PAINS OF THE MENOPAUSE
Menopausal women have to contend with more than just joint pain

CRAMPS
As women get closer to menopause, menstrual cramps are likely to be more severe. This is down to an increased release of a fatty hormone called prostaglandin from the lining of the uterus.

MIGRAINES
Some women know the link between their periods and migraines all too well. Caused by drops in oestrogen, these hormonal headaches are likely to become more frequent and intense as the menopause approaches.

BRUISING
Menopausal women might notice they become more prone to painful bruising. This is because the skin loses its elasticity and ability to retain water – two natural buffers protecting it against injuries.

FIBROMYALGIA
Muscle and joint pain are the hallmarks of fibromyalgia, a condition that intensifies during the menopause. But that's not all – studies show women with menopause symptoms are nearly twice as likely to also have a chronic pain diagnosis.

SEX
Hormonal changes make vaginal tissue thinner, dryer and less stretchy. As a result, sex can become uncomfortable for menopausal women, ranging from a dry, tight feeling in the vagina to severe pains during penetration.

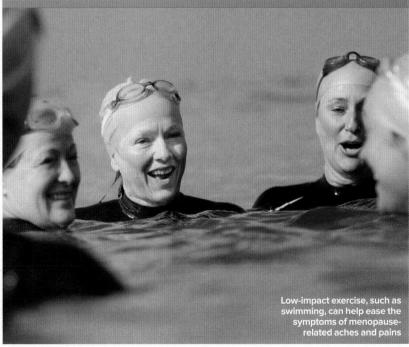

Low-impact exercise, such as swimming, can help ease the symptoms of menopause-related aches and pains

Feeling *Flushed*

The hot flush is one of the most common menopause-related discomforts reported by women. Here's how to cope...

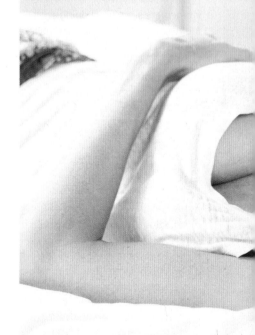

WHAT IS A HOT FLUSH?

A hot flush – also called a hot flash – can be one of the most discomforting ordeals that perimenopausal women experience as they mature. Women describe them as a feeling of heat, growing in intensity, usually starting in the chest or neck and rising to the face. The heat is often – but not in every case – accompanied by a rapid heartbeat or sweating, and the feeling can last from anywhere between one and five minutes before dissipating. After that, many women feel a chill. When experienced during sleep, hot flushes are called night sweats and can severely impair a woman's sleep.

Behind the hot flush is a complex biological event that hasn't been fully studied, so isn't understood by scientists and medical professionals. It's believed that the process starts in the brain, specifically in an area called the hypothalamus, which is a small region that sits right at the centre of the brain. The hypothalamus is responsible for releasing hormones directly into the

"A hot flush varies in length"

bloodstream and has a role in hunger, thirst, tiredness, sleep, sex, and – most relevant to hot flushes – the body's temperature. Though we don't know the exact cause or trigger, we know that the hypothalamus can sense when a person is too warm, and kickstart a chain reaction that cools a person down. The flushed look and feel to a woman's face and neck is caused by blood vessels dilating, which is a method the body uses to cool down and dissipate heat. It can trigger sweating in some women, which is then sometimes followed by a chill as the sweat evaporates off the skin. As you go through the menopause you may begin to notice a pattern to when you begin to flush, but this will be unique to every woman.

HOW LONG DOES A HOT FLUSH LAST?

A hot flush, from that first prickle of heat to the final cooling down period, varies in length for every woman. Typically, it is reported that a hot flush

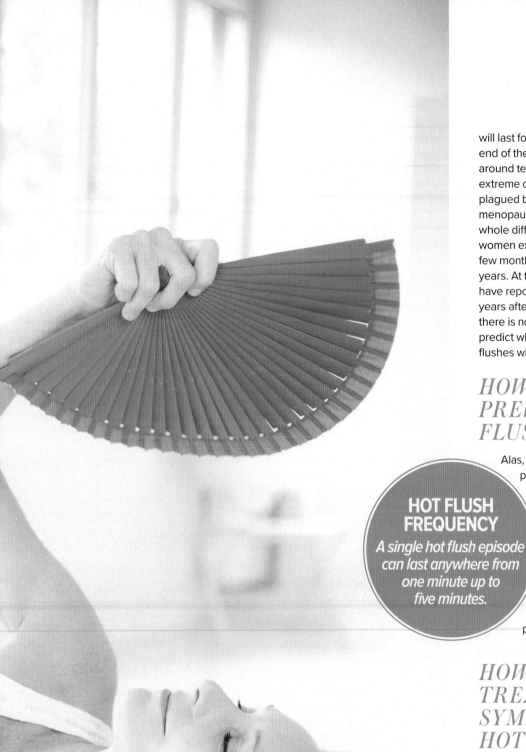

will last for a few minutes, but the top end of the scale seems to hover at around ten minutes in the most extreme cases. How long you will be plagued by hot flushes during your menopause or perimenopause is a whole different question. Some women experience hot flushes for a few months, others for a couple of years. At the extreme, some women have reported hot flushes for up to ten years after menopause. Unfortunately there is no way that anyone can predict when the experience of hot flushes will stop.

HOW CAN YOU PREVENT A HOT FLUSH?

Alas, there is currently no way to prevent a hot flush. We can share advice on how best to manage and treat the uncomfortable feelings caused by hot flushes, but if you find yourself absolutely unable to cope with them, then it is best to seek advice from a medical professional.

HOT FLUSH FREQUENCY

A single hot flush episode can last anywhere from one minute up to five minutes.

HOW CAN YOU TREAT THE SYMPTOMS OF A HOT FLUSH?

You may not be able to stop hot flushes from happening, but you can most definitely find ways to minimise that horrible hot feeling. One of the easiest ways to do so is to be prepared to tackle the symptoms at any time – especially since the onset of a hot flush can't necessarily be predicted. Wear layers of clothes so that you can remove items as necessary to cool down when a hot flush hits you when you're out and about (and then put them back on again later!). It's also worth investing in a paper fan, or a small handheld battery-powered fan. These items are small enough to be put away in a handbag and can be pulled out for

Managing your hot flushes takes time and experimentation. Don't be afraid to try new things in your quest to keep cool

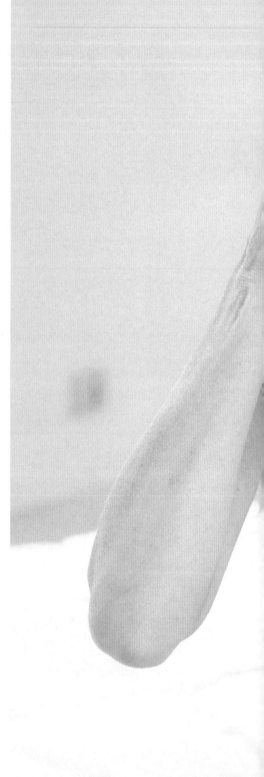

"Ice packs are a quick way to cool the body"

use at your convenience. Cooling facial sprays that are designed to soothe and cool skin during hot weather could come in handy. These are produced and sold by skincare brands in high street drugstores and also online.

Lifestyle changes may also help. Reducing your intake of caffeine, alcohol, and spicy foods (which are thought to be possible triggers) could help alleviate symptoms. Tracking when your hot flushes appear may help you identify possible triggers and therefore the number of flushes that you experience. Tight clothing – especially when worn during hot weather – can exacerbate the creeping heat of a hot flush. Cold compresses and ice packs pressed against veins close to the surface of the skin – inside the elbows, behind the knee, and on the inside of the wrist – are the quickest ways to cool a body down (outside of a cold shower!).

There are certain hormonal and non-hormonal medical treatments that have some success, but they should only come after a discussion with a doctor about your medical history and your symptoms. One non-hormonal treatment is a specific type of antidepressant called an SSRI that can be prescribed to treat hot flushes. Research to find out whether other antidepressants can have a similar effect is currently underway. The dose of the antidepressant is typically low, though it still has a risk of inducing side effects, which may outweigh the benefits. The most common medical treatment is hormonal replacement therapy, called HRT for short. It involves taking a dose of oestrogen

(usually as a gel, spray, or tablet) to replace the oestrogen that your body stops making during menopause. For many women, HRT can relieve a lot of their symptoms.

STAYING HEALTHY AFTER THE MENOPAUSE

You might have found yourself so preoccupied with managing your physical health and mental wellbeing during your period of menopause that you've forgotten what it's like to live without symptoms – but life goes on after the menopause, and soon enough your symptoms will be over and you will be considered to be postmenopausal (having not had a period for more than a year). Your body may have changed now that you have matured beyond the menopause, and maintaining a healthy lifestyle will require a different routine to what you are used to. After menopause, the risks of cancer, diabetes, osteoporosis, and heart disease all rise with age, so it is important to get a yearly check-up with a health professional to catch any potential issues early. Keep track of your height, weight, and blood pressure, all of which can reveal a lot of information about your general health. Discuss with your doctor the need for regular cervical screenings (sometimes called a smear test or pap screen) and mammograms. Unhealthy habits such as smoking, excessive drinking of alcohol, engaging in a sedentary lifestyle, and eating unhealthy foods can all contribute to heart disease, cancer, and diabetes. Menopause is not necessarily responsible for how easy it can be to lose muscle mass at this stage in life – it is mostly related to ageing, which just so happens to come into play after you have become postmenopausal. As ever, you can reduce the risk of developing any of these issues by engaging in regular physical activity, losing excess weight, and maintaining a healthy diet.

COOLING DOWN
To help cool down, wrap a frozen ice pack in a towel and touch it to your neck.

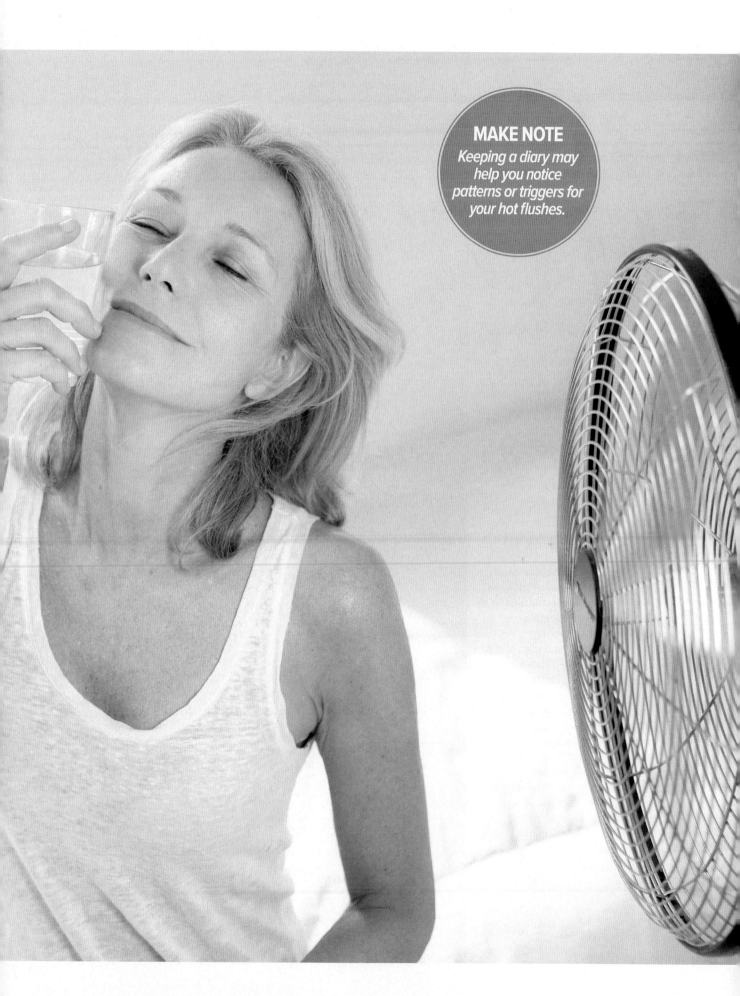

MAKE NOTE
Keeping a diary may help you notice patterns or triggers for your hot flushes.

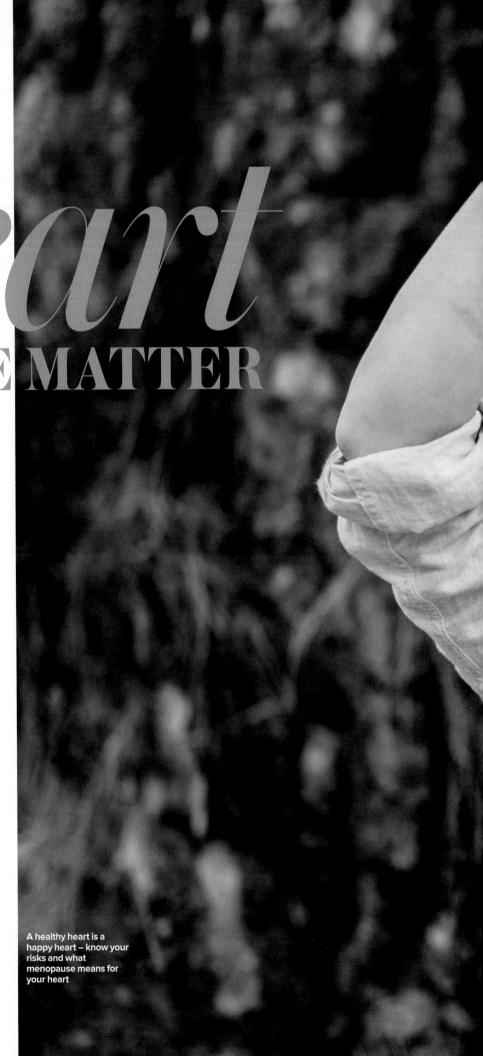

The heart OF THE MATTER

Everything you need to know about heart disease and menopause, and steps to reduce your risk

Words by Ella Carter

Oestrogen – the hormone produced by your ovaries – is primarily responsible for regulating the menstrual cycle. However, we have oestrogen receptors throughout our bodies and it influences a wide range of other areas, which can also begin to change and alter as you enter perimenopause and then eventually menopause. One of these is the impact that decreasing hormone levels can have on your cardiovascular system, which means that women's risk of developing heart disease after menopause is increased. Here you can learn more about why your risk might increase, as well as some things you can easily do to help keep your heart healthy.

A healthy heart is a happy heart – know your risks and what menopause means for your heart

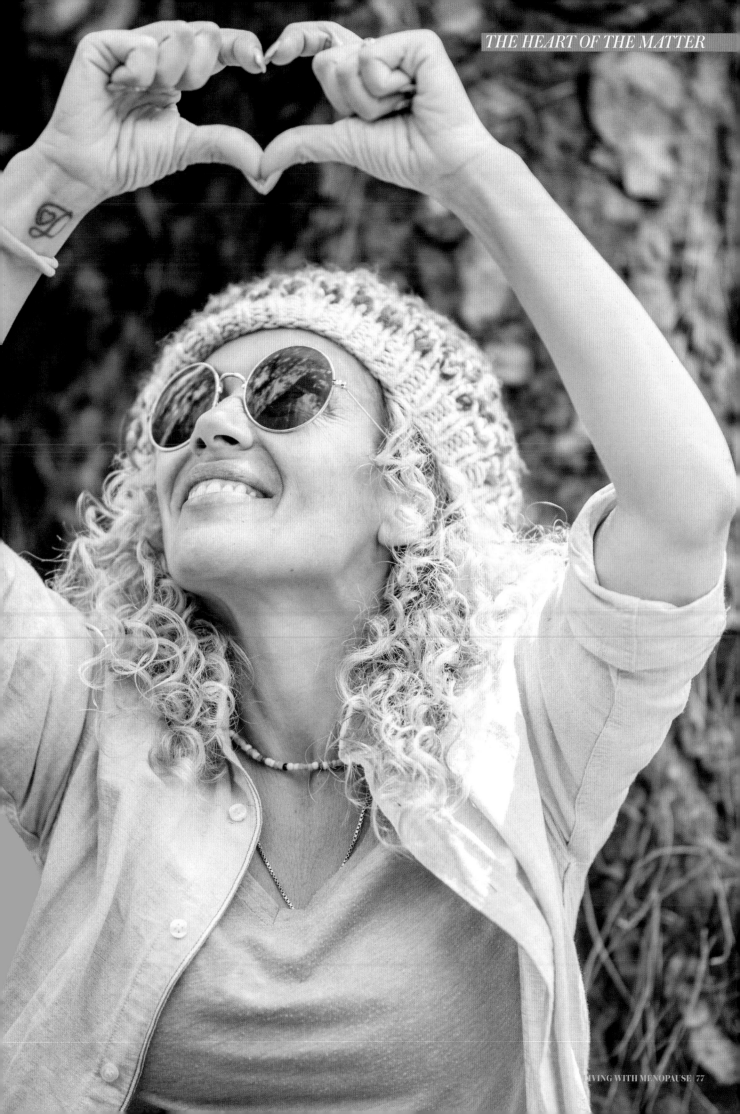

WHAT IS HEART DISEASE AND WHAT CAUSES IT?

The term 'heart disease' is a broad term that's used to describe different conditions that affect the heart or the blood vessels. This is also known as cardiovascular disease (CVD) and is usually associated with a risk of blood clots and the build-up of fatty plaques in the arteries. These factors can reduce the flow of oxygen-rich blood to organs in your body, which if left unchecked,

'Good' cholesterol is called High Density Lipoprotein (or HDL). 'Bad' cholesterol is called Low Density Lipoprotein (LDL, or non-HDL).

can be dangerous and result in heart attack or stroke. However, as with all diseases there are varying levels of severity, and the more you understand about your risk the more steps you can take to help reduce it.

WHAT ARE THE IMPLICATIONS OF GOING THROUGH MENOPAUSE?

It's important to understand that menopause doesn't *cause* heart disease, it just tips the balance of risk and means that you're more vulnerable to developing it.

This is because before menopause, oestrogen plays a role in prevention. It keeps tissues in the body flexible and supple, and has a vasodilative effect, which means it helps keep blood flowing by allowing blood vessels to widen. It also works with your liver to control levels of 'bad' cholesterol (which can cause fatty plaque build-ups on artery walls and cause blockages, leading to heart attacks if levels in your

SYMPTOMS TO LOOK OUT FOR

Visit your doctor for more help and advice if you have any symptoms or are concerned, and in an emergency phone for an ambulance

BREATHLESSNESS
If you feel like you can't catch your breath, or that your breathing is restricted, be sure to seek help.

PALPITATIONS OR IRREGULAR HEARTBEAT
If you feel your heartbeat regularly skipping about, contact your GP for advice. This can be caused by any number of factors but it's always best to be safe!

FATIGUE
This could be due to lifestyle or many other factors, however if you're feeling extremely tired and can't put it down to a specific cause, it's worth checking.

CHEST PAIN
If you're feeling pain in your chest when you're exercising, then check in with your doctor. If you have chest pain and are feeling extremely

unwell, it could be an emergency so phone for an ambulance.

WEAK LIMBS
If you notice that your legs and arms feel weak or you get cramping pains, be sure to mention this to your doctor.

SWOLLEN ANKLES
If you start to notice swelling in your limbs (particularly ankles) then check in with your doctor, as this can be a sign of poor circulation.

FEELING DIZZY OR FAINT
This might be because of low blood pressure, but also other factors. See a doctor to be sure.

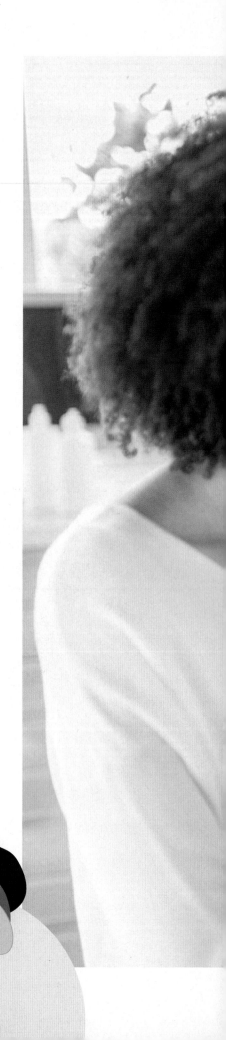

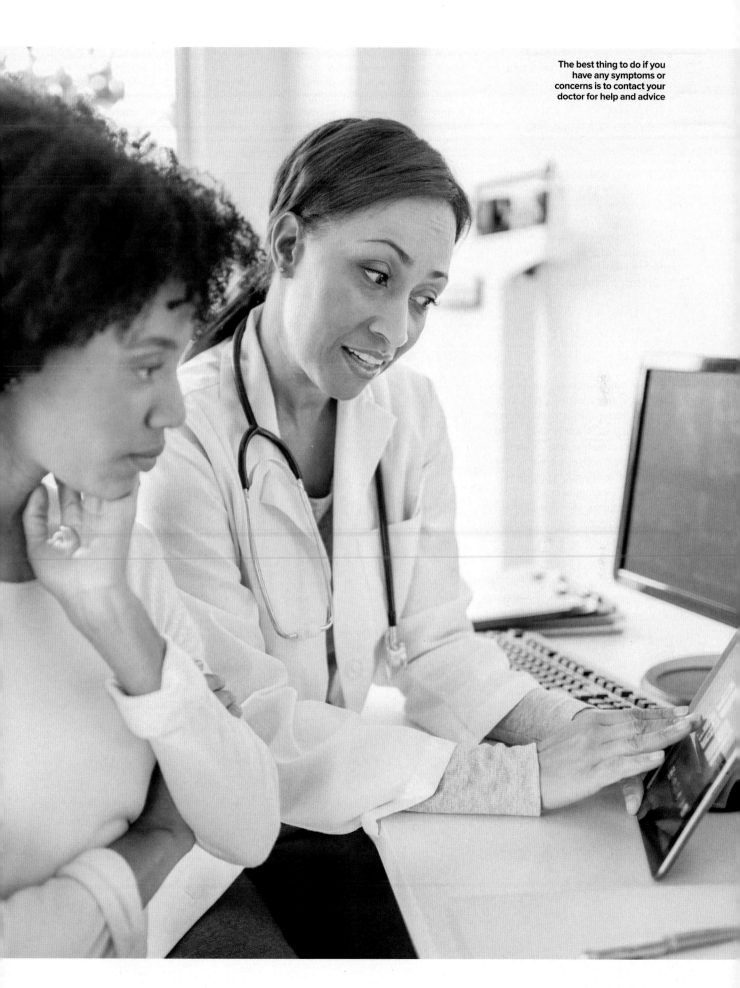

The best thing to do if you have any symptoms or concerns is to contact your doctor for help and advice

body are too high), in addition to promoting more 'good' cholesterol, which contributes to combating the 'bad' cholesterol and keeping blood vessels healthy.

All of these factors mean that a woman's risk of developing heart disease before menopause is lower than a man's. However, at around the average age of 45 when women typically begin to enter perimenopause, this risk begins to rise. This is because the oestrogen in our bodies begins to fall, meaning all of the protective properties start to lessen and cholesterol can start to build up.

HOW IS IT DETECTED AND TREATED?

Talking to your doctor will help you to understand your personal situation best, and your doctor will discuss all kinds of things with you. This will include what to look for, your lifestyle, and understanding and testing any symptoms that you might have. If you are experiencing any symptoms that your doctor thinks will require further consideration and exploration, they may run some diagnostic tests such as blood tests, electrocardiograms (ECGs), scans or X-rays.

If you're diagnosed with heart disease, there are numerous treatments that your doctor might suggest. These range from lifestyle changes, to medication, to surgery if required.

Hormone replacement therapy (HRT) is often offered to women to counter symptoms of the menopause such as hot flushes and night sweats, and there is some evidence to suggest that when taken over time, it can reduce the risk of heart disease. However, there are many different types of HRT and how it's administered, and there are some that

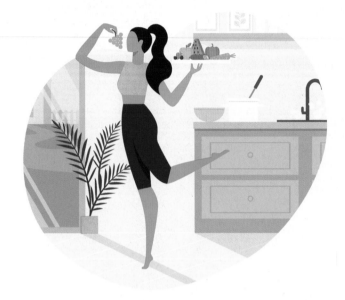

"There are factors that combine with menopause that can put you at a higher susceptibility to developing heart disease"

DIET TIPS FOR A HEALTHY HEART

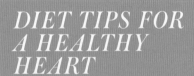
Adapting what you eat is an easy way to ensure you're looking after your heart

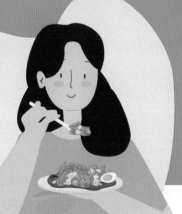

Reduce how much refined sugar you're eating by cutting down on soft drinks, cakes and sweets. This is because sugar can raise blood pressure as well as inflammation.

Eat more oily fish, such as mackerel and sardines. It's full of omega-3, the good fatty acids, which can lower inflammation and help you maintain healthy blood pressure.

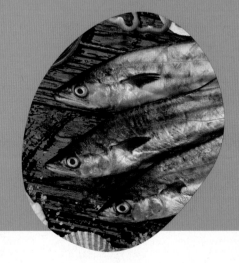

can actually increase the risk of blood clots. It's therefore important that you always talk to your doctor about your personal situation and if you're worried about heart disease or HRT, they'll be able to help you.

WHAT ARE THE RISK FACTORS?

Don't worry – you aren't guaranteed to develop heart disease simply due to the fact that you're going through menopause! It's not a disease that develops for everyone, but the science is there to inform you that the risk is increased once your hormone levels drop, so it's a good idea to take steps where you can to look after your heart. In addition to that, there are some other factors that may combine with menopause that can put you at a higher susceptibility to developing heart disease. Factors such as family history are important to consider. Additionally, if you are overweight or suffer from diabetes, high blood pressure (hypertension) or if you smoke, these are all things that can contribute to a higher risk of heart disease. There are some key steps that you can take in order to help look after your heart, though, no matter your situation! Making some lifestyle changes is something we can all do, to ensure that our hearts are in top shape.

KEY LIFESTYLE CHANGES FOR A HEALTHY HEART

DIET

There are some simple lifestyle changes that you can make to protect your heart, starting with your diet! Avoiding processed foods, trans and saturated fats and adopting a Mediterranean-style diet is the best way to eat your way to heart health. And try to reduce caffeine and alcohol – these are both aggregators of menopause symptoms in general as they can make hot flushes worse, but also important for a healthy ticker. There is a clear link between high blood pressure and alcohol in particular.

EXERCISE

Maintaining your weight is incredibly important for improving blood cholesterol levels and keeping your heart strong and healthy. Exercising regularly can lower your blood pressure, improve blood flow, lower cholesterol and generally reduce your risk of heart disease.
Exercise is also important to support you through menopause as it helps keep your muscles and bones strong as they adapt to the loss of hormones – not to mention the emotional and psychological benefits of exercising!

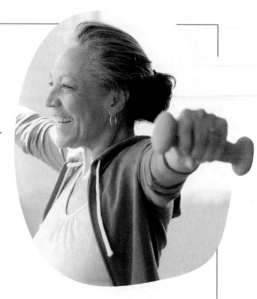

QUIT SMOKING

If you're a smoker, this is one of the biggest things you can do for your health. In addition to increased risk after menopause, smoking seriously increases your risk of heart disease as the chemicals in cigarettes make your arteries sticky, which causes the build-up of plaque to happen more readily. Smoking can also increase your risk of blood clots and instantly increases your blood pressure. If you need help to quit smoking, there are many different support systems out there, or as always, contact your doctor for help and support.

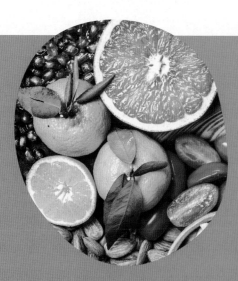

Make sure you get your five-a-day of different colour fruit and veggies – this is to ensure that you have a balance of vitamins, minerals and antioxidants.

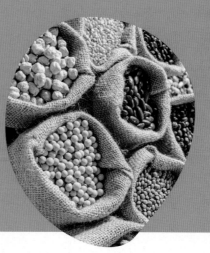

Munch more fibre, as this is good for helping lower cholesterol and blood pressure. Swap white bread for granary, and find fibre in pulses like beans, lentils and chickpeas.

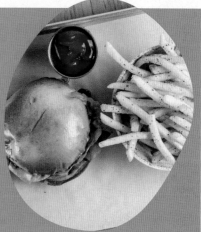

Cut down on trans fats (found in processed foods and takeaways) and saturated fats (from animal products) – these are both known to raise cholesterol.

What's up with your
Hormones?

Understanding the role your hormones play during menopause
can help you navigate the changes you'll be going through
during what can be an emotional time

Words by Lynnette Hecker

Lynnette Hecker *is co-founder of Feeling Flush,
which is dedicated to promoting the fun side of
middle age – facebook.com/feelingflushUK/*

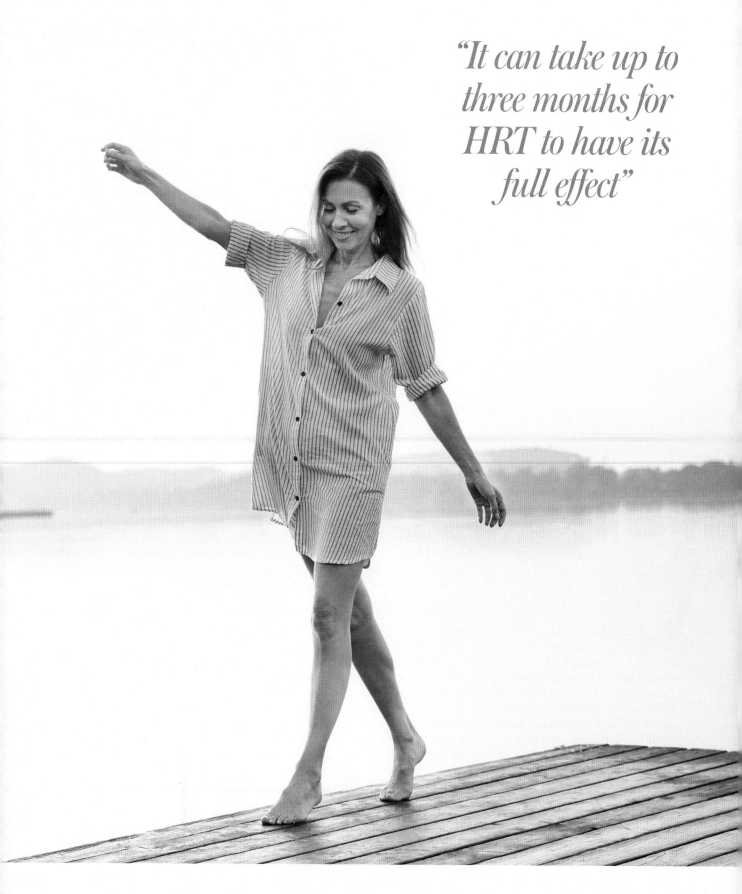

"It can take up to three months for HRT to have its full effect"

Menopause officially starts when it has been 12 months since your last period. The years leading up to this point are called perimenopause. During this stage you might experience changes in your monthly cycle, as well as various physical and emotional symptoms. Any discomfort you feel can be blamed on the declining hormone levels produced by your ovaries as you approach menopause. In fact, hormones are behind pretty much everything to do with the menopause.

Oestrogen, progesterone and testosterone are the main culprits. Produced by the ovaries, they play a key role in the reproductive system when you are younger, only to slow down as you reach the end of your child-bearing years. Without a reproductive system to manage, it makes sense that the body will stop producing the same amount of these hormones. Unfortunately, this decline kicks off menopausal symptoms such as hot flushes, vaginal dryness and brain fog.

EBBING AWAY OF OESTROGEN

Ovaries produce oestrogen in the reproductive years, but during menopause, the ovaries no longer do this. Oestrogen is one of the main female hormones and is essential for the growth and health of reproductive organs. It affects sexual function as it maintains the flow of blood in the vagina, vaginal elasticity and lubrication. It also causes the lining of the uterus to thicken during the menstrual cycle. Oestrogen not only helps with brain function, heart and bone health and cholesterol, but it keeps the lining of the bladder in good condition.

Once these levels start to fluctuate, physical changes occur. Low levels of oestrogen can lead to hot flushes, night sweats, heart palpitations, headaches, insomnia, fatigue, bone loss and vaginal dryness.

The dropping of oestrogen levels as women near menopause can also

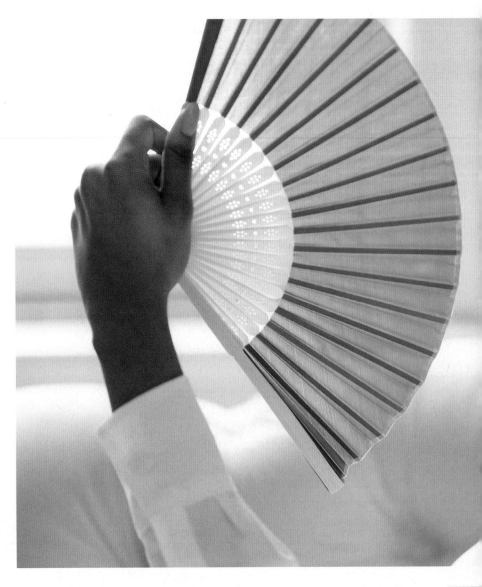

cause pelvic muscles to weaken. This in turn can lead to some women losing bladder control. According to the NHS, as many as 70 percent of women relate the onset of their urinary incontinence to their final menstrual period. Losing weight, cutting down on caffeine and alcohol, doing pelvic floor exercises and bladder training can all help.

Eating a plant-based diet can also be of more general help, as oestrogen is naturally present in various foods such as dried fruits, vegetables, soy products, pulses and lentils, flaxseed and different herbs.

THE PART PLAYED BY PROGESTERONE

Progesterone is the other main female hormone – it's a steroid hormone released by the corpus luteum (a normal cyst that forms on the ovary

every month in women of childbearing age) to stimulate the uterus. It prepares the lining of the uterus for a fertilised egg and helps maintain early pregnancy. Intermittent reductions of this hormone in perimenopause can mean irregular, heavier or longer periods. When it comes to postmenopause, the significantly reduced level of progesterone means skin no longer maintains its elasticity and you can experience vaginal dryness, water retention and bloating. Increasing your intake of vitamins B and C and eating food with zinc (such as shellfish) can help.

TESTOSTERONE TALES

Testosterone in women is essential for the development and maintenance of female sexual anatomy. It peaks when women are in their 20s and then

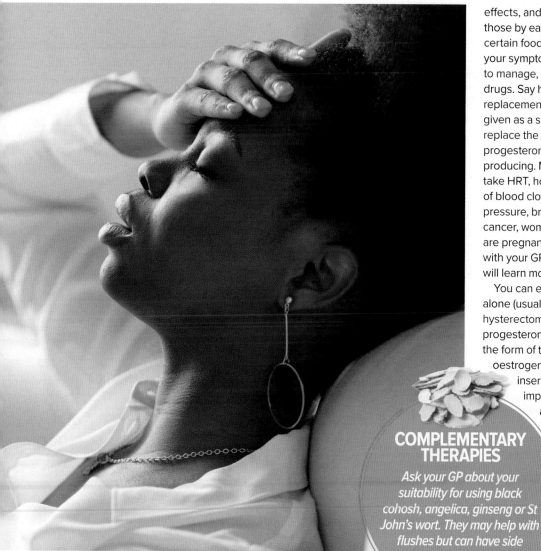

effects, and you can try to counter those by eating certain foods, avoiding certain foods and exercising. But if your symptoms are proving impossible to manage, it may be time for some drugs. Say hello to hormonal replacement therapy (HRT). This is given as a supplementary hormone to replace the oestrogen and progesterone your body stops producing. Most women are able to take HRT, however if you have a history of blood clots, untreated high blood pressure, breast cancer, ovarian cancer, womb cancer, liver disease or are pregnant, you will need to consult with your GP about alternatives (you will learn more about these later).

You can either take just oestrogen alone (usually if you've had a hysterectomy) or both oestrogen and progesterone together. This can be in the form of tablets, skin patches, an oestrogen gel or vaginal cream, or inserting a pessary, ring or implant. All have their own advantages. Tablets are the most common form of HRT and can be taken daily, although patches can help avoid some side effects of HRT, such as indigestion. Gel can also be rubbed on once a day, while implants release oestrogen gradually and can last for a few months, but they are not widely used. Vaginal oestrogen can help locally but does not address other symptoms.

COMPLEMENTARY THERAPIES

Ask your GP about your suitability for using black cohosh, angelica, ginseng or St John's wort. They may help with flushes but can have side effects with other medications.

declines very slowly after that. This is caused by both age and ovarian function. There is still a debate about whether the dampening of libido because of lower testosterone levels is due to menopause or age. By the time you reach menopause, though, testosterone levels are half of what they were at their peak. If you find you are suffering because of this, testosterone can be rubbed on the skin in gel form, but is currently only available via specialist doctors rather than the NHS. Side effects can include acne and unwanted hair growth.

MAKING UP FOR LOST HORMONES

So, we know that a decline in hormone levels can bring on a tsunami of menopausal symptoms and side

RISKS OF TAKING HRT

The benefits of taking HRT generally outweigh any risks but this will depend on your age and health, how long you take it for and the type of treatment. Always speak to a GP to find out all the latest information.

Taking HRT tablets carries a small risk of blood clots, as oestrogen can cause platelets in the blood to clump, but patches and gels don't. Taking HRT tablets is also linked to a very small possibility of stroke, although the British Heart Foundation says that women taking HRT do not have a higher risk of dying from a stroke or a

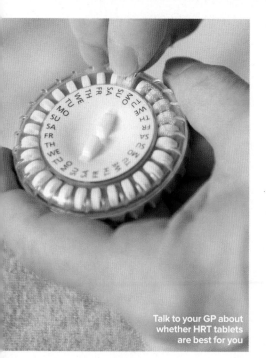

Talk to your GP about whether HRT tablets are best for you

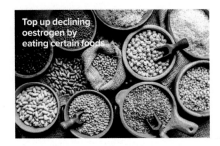

Top up declining oestrogen by eating certain foods

heart attack than women who have never taken it.

It's important to note that HRT can take up to three months to have its full effect. It can cause side effects in the first three months of use, but these vary between women. Talk to your GP about changing the type or dose you are on if you are still experiencing symptoms after three months.

One of the most publicised side effects of HRT, though, is breast cancer. Research into whether there is a link between taking HRT and getting breast cancer has changed over the years. Up until 2002, all the research pointed to HRT being safe to use, but then a Women's Health Initiative (WHI) study found it increased the risk in women taking combined HRT (oestrogen and progesterone). When that study was looked at again, it was found to show that there were just an extra eight cases of breast cancer for every 10,000 women taking HRT for a year. Current thinking is that for most women under the age of 60, HRT benefits outweigh any negatives. The NHS says there is little or no change in the risk of breast cancer if you take oestrogen-only HRT. Combined HRT can be associated with a small increase in the risk of breast cancer, however this is related to how long you take it, and reduces after you stop taking it.

HOW LONG DO YOU NEED TO TAKE HRT FOR?

The menopause does not stop when you start taking HRT and then start when you stop taking it. It purely alleviates symptoms.

There are no limits on how long you can take HRT. Generally, it is taken for two to three years but it is advisable to speak to your GP about what is best for you. Gradually decreasing your HRT dose is recommended because it means it is less likely that symptoms return in the short-term.

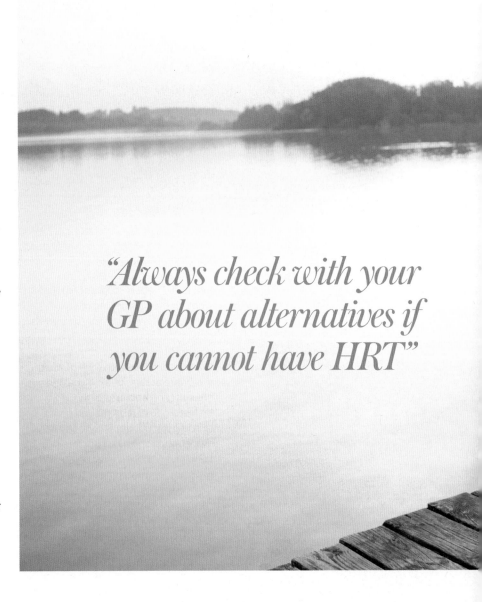

"Always check with your GP about alternatives if you cannot have HRT"

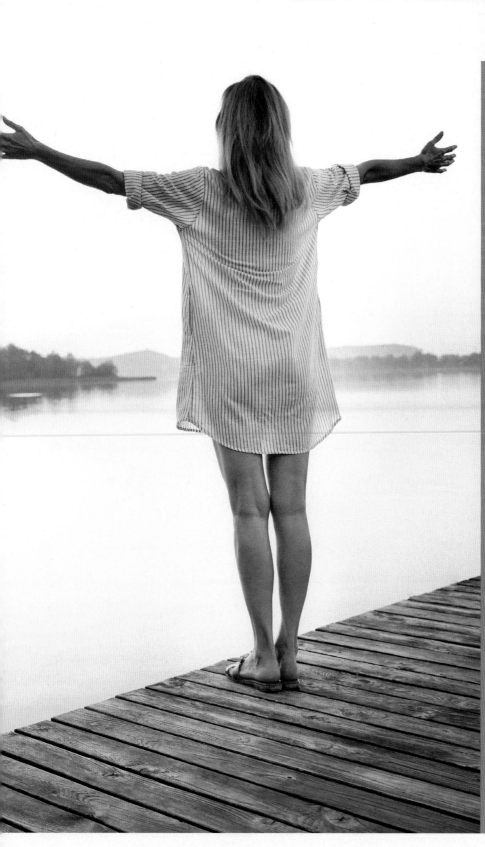

IF YOU CAN'T HAVE *HRT*

Sometimes a GP will not recommend HRT if you have a history of breast, ovarian or womb cancer, in addition to other health conditions. But that doesn't mean you have to suffer. There are alternatives...

COGNITIVE BEHAVIOURAL THERAPY (CBT)

CBT can be helpful for menopause if symptoms include anxiety, stress, mood swings and irritability. It helps deal with negative thoughts you may have about yourself and your actions.

ANTIDEPRESSANTS

Talk to your GP if you feel depressed. Some antidepressants can help with mood issues but are not considered as the first line of treatment. However, they may help with hot flushes if you are not able to take oestrogen.

HOT FLUSH MEDICINES

A blood pressure medication called clonidine and an epilepsy medicine called gabapentin are both thought to help with hot flushes. Neither affect hormone levels, so talk to your GP about if they would be useful.

BIOIDENTICAL OR 'NATURAL HORMONES'

These are made from plant sources that are converted into hormone preparations and are said to be similar to human hormones. However, the NHS does not currently recommend them as they are not regulated.

SELF-CARE FOR PERIMENOPAUSE:

Where a little self-love goes a long way

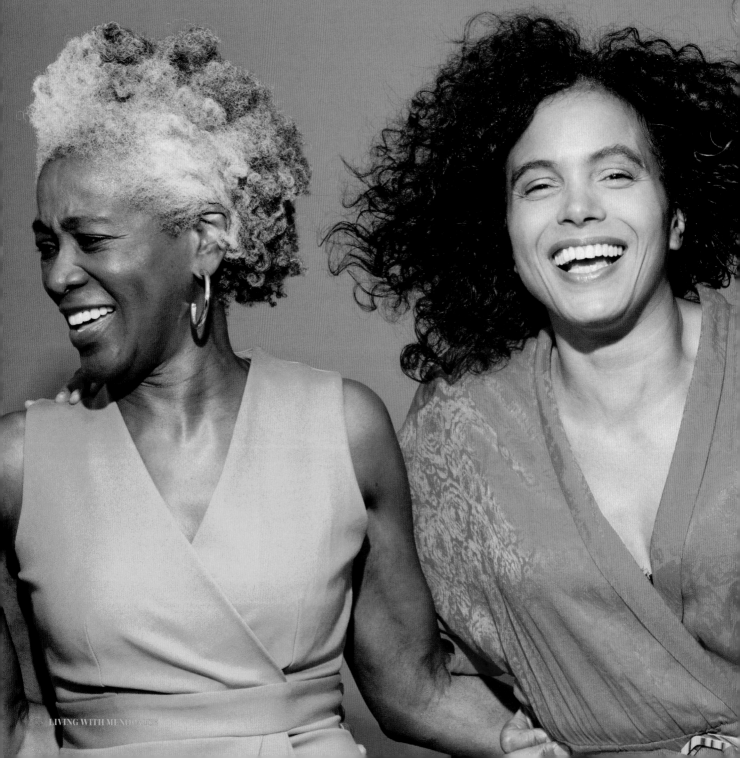

Simple steps to boost vitality, confidence and improve most perimenopause symptoms

Words by Kate Codrington

Perimenopause may start earlier than you think. It can even show up in your late 30s with changes to your periods, energy or mood. You'll be surprised what a difference small tweaks to your diet, exercise and self-care routine can make to your symptoms. We're not talking radical change because life is stressful enough already! Small shifts are far more sustainable that will grow into bigger changes over time and pave the way for a vibrant postmenopause life.

◆ **Second Spring: the self-care guide to menopause**, named one of the 10 best self-help books of 2022 by The Independent, is published by HarperCollins and is available to buy for £14.99.

second spring
The self-care guide to menopause
kate codrington

STAY COOL

Hot flushes range from barely noticeable to utterly debilitating. It's the changes in hormone balance that are thought to cause this and managing them needs a multi-layered approach. Start by tracking likely triggers, such as alcohol, sugar, spicy food and caffeine to find how you might reduce their impact. Stress is a major factor in hormone balance, so building in micro-moments of calm throughout your day will help, even taking a few breaths in the bathroom can be a life-saver. At work, flushes can completely derail us because at their height, coherent thought just vanishes! Being honest with co-workers and your boss about what's happening helps to reduce your tension. By naming and accepting what's happening yourself, you're also giving your colleagues permission to talk about their own peri-challenges, so you're doing everyone a favour.

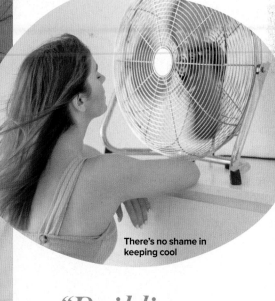

There's no shame in keeping cool

"Building in micro-moments of calm can help"

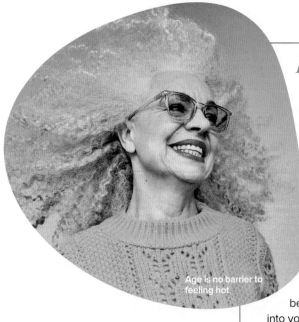

Age is no barrier to feeling hot

FEEL HOT!

It's not always true that our sex-drive tanks at perimenopause, it's just we need something different to turn us on. As your body is changing, it is easy to get out of date with what gives you pleasure, so the first step is to discover for yourself what your body needs and then, if you want to, communicate this with a partner. Pleasuring yourself helps you relax, sleep well, and by improving circulation to the area, supports health and lubrication too. We may not be as juicy as we used to be but lube is a great ally – just check it's free of glycerine, glycol and parabens. Our vulvas need special care. Steer clear of bath bombs, perfumed soap and feminine washes. Pain should always be taken seriously, so go to your physician if you experience any pain. Topical oestrogen is easily available and has minimal dosage. The best thing you can do is to de-stress by building small pleasures into your life. Giving yourself tiny sensual delights each day will shift your dial towards the right kind of hot.

"We need to reduce agitation by building more calm into our lives"

SWEET DREAMS

Sleep deprivation is torture. When dealing with the combination of brain fog and exhaustion, just dragging yourself through your day without major mishap can be a miracle. Unfortunately no one pill or supplement will fix your sleep. We need to look at the bigger picture and reduce agitation by slowing down and building more calm into our lives. Mindfulness can take many forms, so do it your way: a quiet cup of tea, meditation app, stroking your pet or being in nature are all great. Naps in the daytime can help you feel better rested when they are not too close to bedtime. Affirming your circadian rhythm is helpful too. Make sure you get outside in daylight as early as possible in the morning, and at the end of your day, put away phones and laptops a few hours before bed.

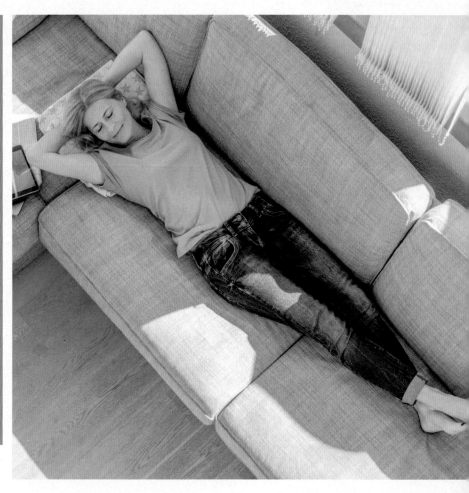

Resting is essential in perimenopause

GOOD MOOD

As our hormones bounce up and down like ping pong balls in perimenopause, our mood can bounce around too, sometimes to extremes, especially in the second half of your menstrual cycle. A time of increased sensitivity, it is vital you prioritise your mental health at perimenopause and give yourself as much me-time as you possibly can. No guilt here. Unfortunately you can find yourself longing for more space right at the point when you have more responsibilities than ever. Call in whatever activity you've enjoyed in the past and probably ditched because you had no time: yoga, walking in nature, reading, dancing, maybe singing? Book it into your diary as a non-negotiable. If you find it hard to give this to yourself, remember that unless you fulfill yourself, you will not be able to serve the people you need to, and by giving to yourself first you are teaching them good self-care too: win-win!

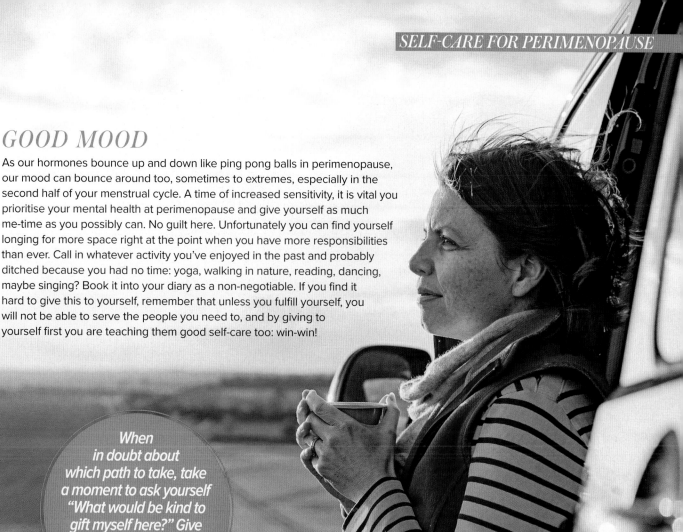

When in doubt about which path to take, take a moment to ask yourself "What would be kind to gift myself here?" Give yourself a regular micro-dose of what you long for.

Taking time for yourself is priceless

HAPPY BODY

Move in a way that feels good for you!

It's true that we can carry a little more weight round our middles in perimenopause, and we can find that reducing calories and exercising no longer has the magic effect it used to. The reason it's hard to shift is because hormone fluctuations make us more sensitive to stress and this piles the weight on, even when you eat fewer calories and exercise hard. Perimenopause is asking us to be kind to ourselves: reduce the amount of stress in our lives and manage it better, eat as healthily as we are able to. Instead of dieting, perhaps it's time to see if you are eating to cover some uncomfortable emotions. So much of our eating is driven by childhood patterns but by identifying our feelings and tending to them, we can make healthier food choices more easily.

Images: Getty Images

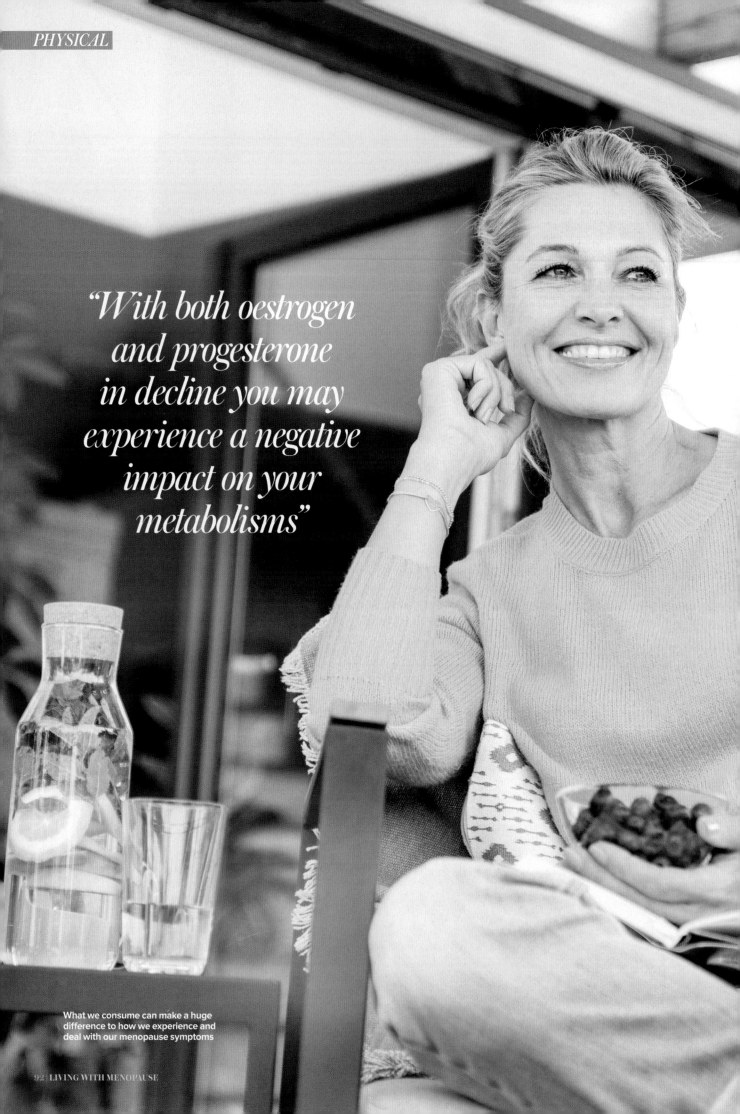

"*With both oestrogen and progesterone in decline you may experience a negative impact on your metabolisms*"

What we consume can make a huge difference to how we experience and deal with our menopause symptoms

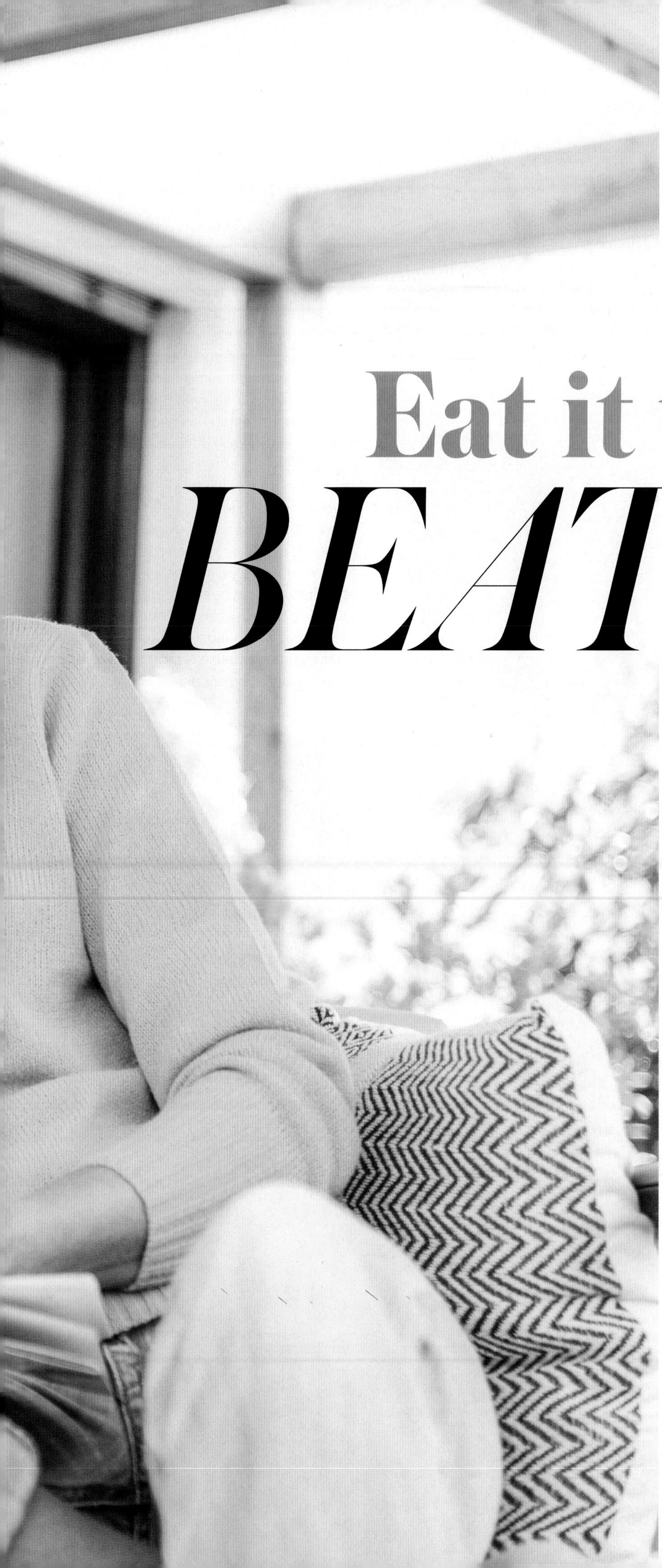

Eat it to
BEAT IT

By making some
dietary changes,
you may be able to
relieve many of your
menopause symptoms

Words by Bee Ginger

As your body embarks on its
journey through the
menopause and beyond, you
lose the ability to produce as much
of the hormone oestrogen as you
did during your menstrual cycles.
With both oestrogen and progesterone
in decline, you may experience a
negative impact on your metabolisms,
often leading to weight gain, the
inability to properly digest
carbohydrates, and varying levels of
cholesterol. These hormonal changes
can also lead to a decline in your bone
density, which in turn can increase the
risk of bone fractures. This is in
addition to all the other menopausal
joys, such as insomnia and hot flushes.

Your menopause is linked to many
varied symptoms and can also increase
your risk of differing diseases.
However, by taking a closer look at
your diet and making a few simple
changes, you may be able to reduce
your menopause symptoms and
transition into the next stage with ease.

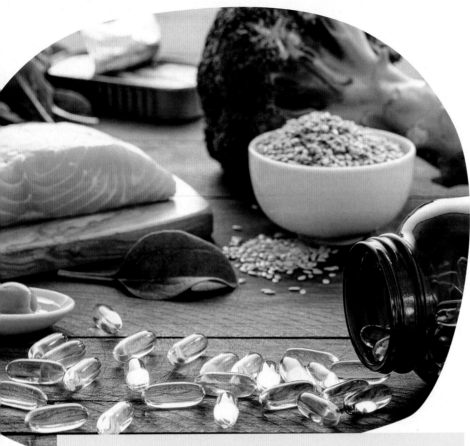

WHOLE GRAINS

Diets high in whole grains are not just beneficial during the menopause but have been linked to a reduction in the risk of both cancer and heart disease. Whole grains are packed full of nutrients, fibre, pantothenic acid, riboflavin, thiamine and niacin. Good sources of whole grain include whole wheat bread, quinoa, rye, barley and brown rice. Research has uncovered that people regularly consuming three or more servings of whole grains each day have a greatly lowered risk of developing diabetes and heart disease when compared to those regularly eating more refined carbohydrates, such as white bread and rice. Fibre is essential in aiding healthy digestion, balancing blood sugar, regulating cholesterol, and – most importantly during the menopause – promoting a good hormonal balance.

HEALTHY FATS

Our bodies benefit greatly from an increase in fatty acids such as omega-3. The most omega-3-rich foods include seeds like chia, flax and hemp, as well as fatty fish like anchovies, mackerel and salmon. These fatty acids may also be a benefit to women going through the menopause and are said to assist in decreasing the severity and frequency of both night sweats and hot flushes. If you are not a fan of eating fish you can always take an omega-3 supplement, which has also been proven to be beneficial. Fatty fish and omega-3 fatty acids are the key to improving not just bone health but also mood and brain function. They also keep blood pressure levels in check, which in turn helps control the hot flushes.

DAIRY PRODUCTS

As oestrogen levels decline during menopause, there is an increased risk of bone fractures. Women therefore benefit greatly from consuming dairy products like yoghurt, milk and cheese, which contain essential vitamins and minerals for bone health, including vitamin K, magnesium, vitamin D, phosphorus, potassium and good old calcium. Studies have found that women who consumed more dairy during the menopause had a far higher bone density than those who hadn't increased their consumption. Furthermore, both cheese and milk contain high levels of the amino acid glycine, which promotes better sleep. Another great reason for a hot chocolate before bed!

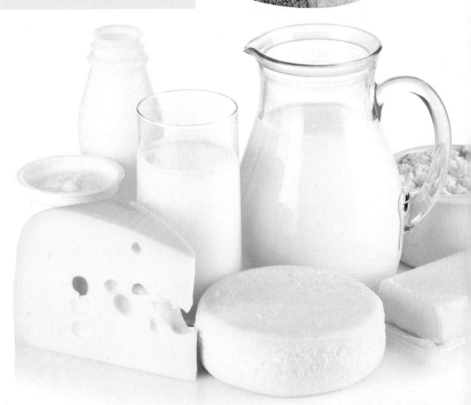

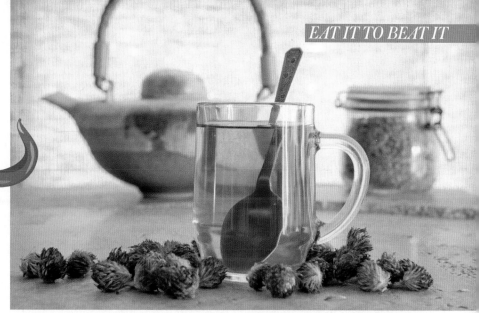

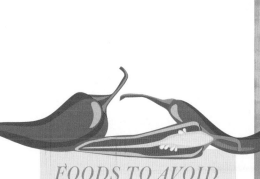

FOODS TO AVOID

Many sources suggest that women avoid spicy foods while going through the menopause. Spicy foods can make your hot flushes worse, particularly foods containing cayenne, hot peppers and other hot spices. Alcohol can also exacerbate your flushes and interfere with your sleep. However, your reaction to food is as individual as you are, so experiment and use your best judgement when including certain foods in your diet. If your menopausal symptoms, worsen then cut them out.

HIGH-QUALITY PROTEIN

We have already learned that when bodies commence their journey through the menopause, they suffer a decline in oestrogen. This decline, however, is linked to a decrease in both bone strength and muscle mass. Therefore we need to increase our consumption of protein. We can find this in dairy products, eggs, meat, fish, nuts, seeds and legumes, all of which are fantastic sources of protein. You can even buy a range of protein powders to add to your morning smoothie for that added boost.

Foods rich in protein are often more filling than other foods and take longer to digest. This gives your body a steadier supply of energy and you will find you are less likely to crave carbohydrate-rich or sugary foods later on in the day. By eating plenty of protein you can help your body to maintain a healthy muscle mass and a good metabolism. This can also help limit menopausal weight gain, as a good metabolism and healthy muscles will burn more calories.

FOODS RICH IN PHYTOESTROGEN

Research suggests that phytoestrogens may have health benefits, particularly for women journeying through the menopause. The compounds found in phytoestrogens act as weak oestrogens in the body and are naturally found in foods such as chickpeas, flax seeds, grapes, berries, black and green tea, barley, plums and soybeans, to name a few. Studies have shown that phytoestrogens actually help to lower the intensity of hot flushes. Other phytoestrogens aid sleep and cognition, decrease vaginal dryness and improve bone health.

And while we're on the subject of bones, studies have shown that a high intake of salt is linked to a lower bone density in post-menopausal women. Therefore by reducing your intake of sodium, you may be able to lower this risk. Studies have also shown that women who moderated their intake of sodium benefitted from a better overall mood.

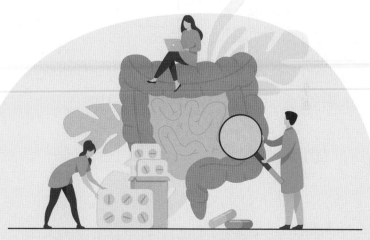

GOOD GUT HEALTH

We know that oestrogen is essential for reproductive health, but it is fundamental that we have balanced and healthy oestrogen for gut health as well. Healthy oestrogen levels ensure that gut barrier integrity is maintained, in addition to promoting the growth of beneficial bacteria and decreasing inflammation in the body. When the body lacks enough oestrogen, the vagina and urethra's tissue lining often becomes thin, dry and inflamed. Many women journeying through the menopause experience dryness, which leads to painful intercourse, yeast and urinary tract infections, bacterial vaginosis and incontinence. Thankfully, by looking at diet and eating to promote a healthy balance of good gut bacteria, it is possible to reduce these symptoms. Phytoestrogens, ground flax seeds, vegetables and fruit are all key to good gut health.

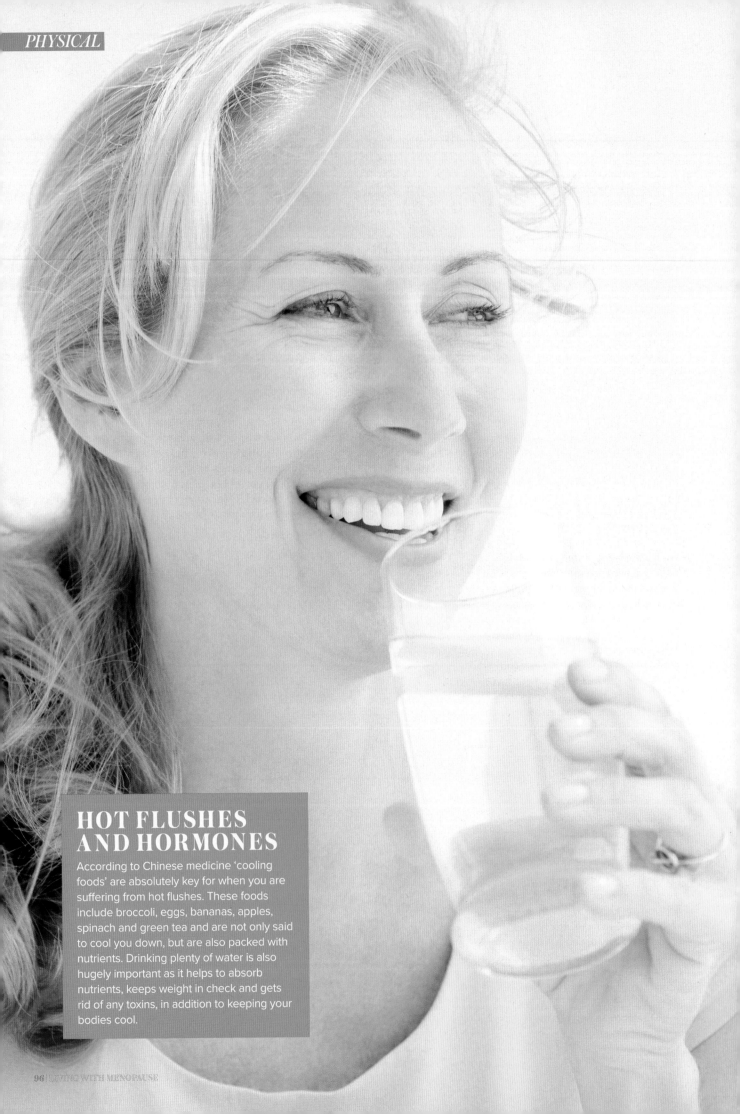

HOT FLUSHES AND HORMONES

According to Chinese medicine 'cooling foods' are absolutely key for when you are suffering from hot flushes. These foods include broccoli, eggs, bananas, apples, spinach and green tea and are not only said to cool you down, but are also packed with nutrients. Drinking plenty of water is also hugely important as it helps to absorb nutrients, keeps weight in check and gets rid of any toxins, in addition to keeping your bodies cool.

SEED CYCLING

Your hormones can be your best friend or your worst enemy, sometimes leaving you with the feeling that they and your body are conspiring against you. Hormones control emotions, moods, sleep, energy and reproduction, to mention just a few things. They are incredibly sophisticated and need to be in perfect balance to work properly. A natural way to balance them can be achieved through seed cycling.

Rooted in naturopathic philosophy, this process matches different seeds to different phases of your hormonal cycle to add nourishment. Seed cycling can provide support in alleviating symptoms associated with declining levels of progesterone and oestrogen during menopause, and can even help to minimise hormonal fluctuations and mood swings, improve sleep quality and energy levels, and reduce hot flushes. Not only can seeds balance your hormones but they are full of antioxidants, minerals and vitamins, not to mention being a great source of both fibre and protein. They are even good for your skin and hair. Seeds are an easy addition to your meals and can taste great in porridge, yoghurt, salads and soups.

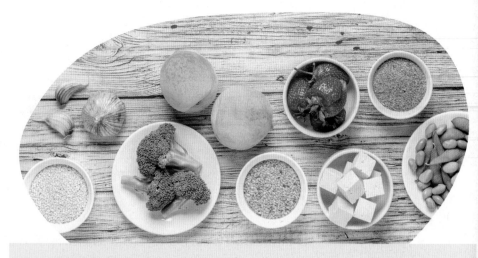

STRIKING THE RIGHT BALANCE

What you consume can make a huge difference in how you experience menopausal symptoms. By being more mindful of what you eat, you are able to better protect your vital organs and bones by consuming the right amount of nutrients.

Vegetables and fruit are integral in any diet, with so many rich in powerful antioxidants that help to prevent cell damage. It's not just the green, leafy vegetables like kale, spinach and broccoli that are needed but also aubergine, carrots, tomatoes, peppers, berries, mangos and cherries, all of which are rich in antioxidants.

"Seed cycling can help minimise hormonal fluctuations, mood swings and reduce hot flushes"

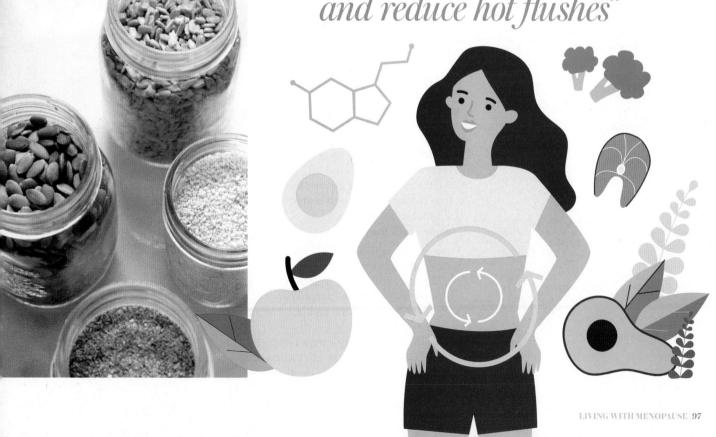

Happy Hormone
RECIPES

Delicious recipes to help balance your hormones,
beat fatigue and lift your mood

ENERGISING SPRING BREAK SHAKE

MAKES 1 SERVING

- **2 large handfuls of spinach**
- **Avocado (or 2 tablespoons raw cashews)**
- **1-inch chunk fresh ginger (or 1 tablespoon dried ginger)**
- **1 scoop vegan unflavoured or vanilla protein powder**
- **1 tablespoon ground flaxseed**
- **Fresh juice of ¹/₂ lemon (or lime)**
- **¹/₂ tablespoon raw apple cider vinegar**
- **1¹/₂ cups plain coconut water or filtered water**
- **Handful of ice (optional)**

OPTIONAL TOPPINGS:

- **Broccoli sprouts and/or extra lemon**

Add all ingredients to a blender. Blend until smooth.

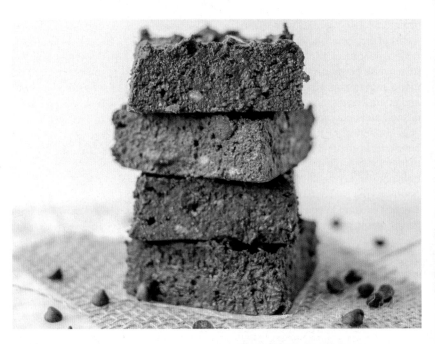

SWEET FUDGY FLOURLESS FEEL-BETTER BROWNIES

MAKES 8 BROWNIES

- **2 medium-sized ripe bananas, mashed**
- **2 tablespoons runny almond butter (can sub any nut or seed butter)**
- **2 tablespoons unsweetened apple sauce (can sub for almond butter)**
- **¹/₂ cup raw cacao powder**
- **1 scoop vegan protein powder (chocolate or vanilla)**
- **2 tablespoons vegan chocolate chips, plus more for topping**

Preheat oven to 180C / 350F / gas mark 4. Whisk the mashed bananas, almond butter and apple sauce in a large bowl. Stir in the cacao powder and protein powder and mix until completely smooth. Stir in the chocolate chips.

Line a loaf pan with parchment paper or grease it with coconut oil and then transfer the batter into the pan. You'll find it will be very thick — use a spatula to spread it out evenly.

Sprinkle extra chocolate chips on top. Bake for 20-25 minutes. The brownies will seem underdone when you take them out, but they will firm up after cooling. Once cool, slice into eight squares.

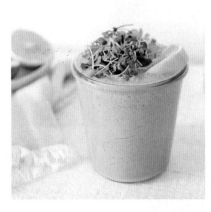

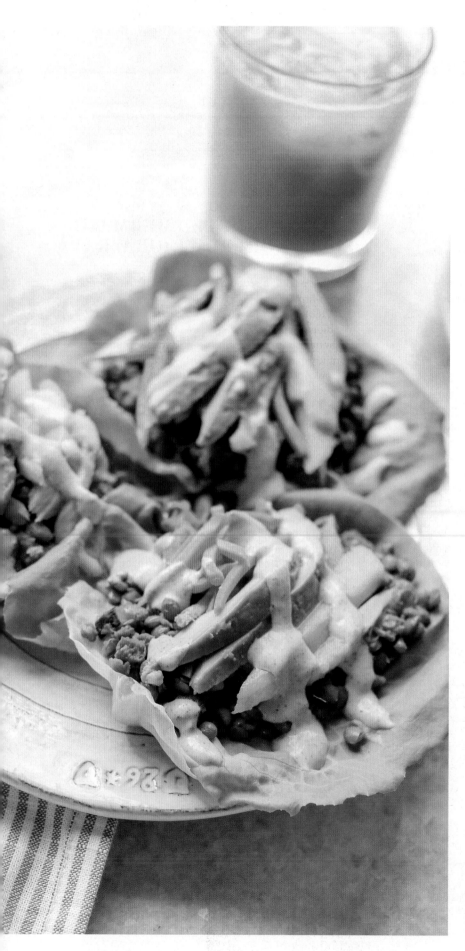

SPRING LENTIL LETTUCE CUPS

MAKES 2 SERVINGS

- **1 cup uncooked green lentils**
- **2 cups filtered water**
- **1 tablespoon coconut oil or avocado oil**
- **¹/₃ white onion, chopped**
- **¹/₂ jalapeño, optional**
- **1 cup courgette/zucchini (finely diced)**
- **1 tablespoon paprika**
- **¹/₂ teaspoon sea salt**
- **¹/₂ tablespoon raw apple cider vinegar**
- **1 ripe mango, cubed**
- **1 cup shredded carrots**
- **Butter lettuce**

OPTIONAL TOPPINGS:

- **Vegan Hemp Ranch (recipe below), sliced avocado, pumpkin seeds, broccoli sprouts, raw sauerkraut**
- **Try serving these lettuce cups with guava kombucha, as pictured.**

In a medium-sized pot, combine lentils with water and bring to a boil, then reduce heat to simmer for 15-20 minutes, or until water is absorbed and lentils are soft. In a separate small saucepan, heat the oil on medium-high heat and sauté the onion, occasionally stirring for 3-4 minutes. Add the jalapeño, courgette/zucchini, paprika and sea salt, and cook for 8-9 minutes, or until courgette/zucchini softens. Turn off heat and stir in apple cider vinegar. Assemble each lettuce cup with lentils, mango, shredded carrot, avocado and optional Vegan Hemp Ranch.

VEGAN HEMP RANCH

MAKES 3-4 SERVINGS

- **¹/₃ cup hemp hearts**
- **¹/₃ cup raw cashews**
- **2 tablespoons extra virgin olive oil**
- **1¹/₂ tablespoons raw apple cider vinegar**
- **1 clove garlic**
- **1 teaspoon sea salt**
- **1 teaspoon dried dill (or 1 tablespoon fresh dill)**
- **1 handful fresh parsley**
- **1 tablespoon chopped green onion**
- **¹/₂ cup filtered water**

In a small blender or a food processor, combine all the ingredients and blend until smooth and creamy. If it's too thick, add 1-2 tablespoons water until you reach the desired consistency.

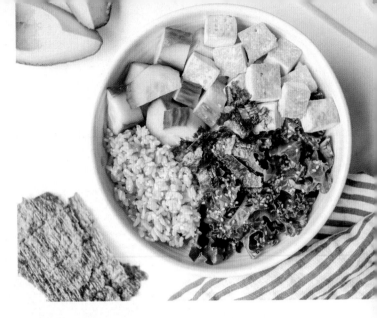

MASHED VEGGIE 'POTATOES' WITH CHEESY BRUSSELS SPROUTS AND KALE

MAKES 2-3 SERVINGS

- **454 g / 1 lb brussels sprouts**, stems removed and halved
- **2 tablespoons avocado oil**
- **1 tablespoon nutritional yeast**
- **1 teaspoon red pepper flakes**
- **Pinch of sea salt**
- **1 rutabaga, peeled and cubed** (can substitute for 2 parsnips)
- **1 turnip, peeled and cubed** (can substitute for 2 parsnips)
- **1/2 head cauliflower florets**
- **Splash of plain unsweetened almond milk** (or any plain nut milk)
- **1 tablespoon refined coconut oil**
- **Sea salt, to taste**
- **2 cups chopped kale leaves**

OPTIONAL ADD-INS:
- **Chickpeas**

Preheat oven to 200C / 400F / gas mark 6. Line a baking sheet with parchment paper. Toss brussels sprouts with oil, nutritional yeast, red pepper flakes, and sea salt. Roast for 20-25 minutes or until crispy.

Meanwhile, bring a large pot filled with water to a boil. After the water boils, add rutabaga, turnip, and cauliflower. Boil for 20 minutes or until the veggies are tender.

While the vegetables are boiling, steam kale in a pan or small pot fitted with a steamer basket for about five minutes. When veggies are soft, drain well and add them back into the large pot with almond milk, coconut oil, and sea salt. Mash with a potato masher or a hand immersion blender.

Assemble your plate with mashed 'potatoes,' cheesy Brussels sprouts, and steamed kale.

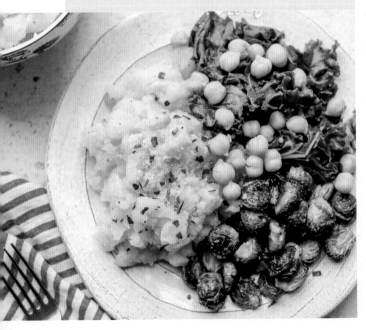

DECONSTRUCTED MERMAID SUSHI NORI BOWL (OR WRAP)

MAKES 2 SERVINGS

- **1 14-oz package organic extra-firm tofu**
- **2-4 tablespoons low-sodium tamari** (to marinate tofu) or liquid aminos
- **2 tablespoons rice vinegar, divided**
- **1/2 cup uncooked short-grain brown rice** (or 1 cup cooked)
- **1/2 cucumber, chopped**
- **4 cups kale, chopped** (can sub spinach)
- **1 tablespoon maple syrup**
- **1 avocado, cubed**
- **1–2 large nori seaweed sheets** (or dulse flakes)

OPTIONAL TOPPINGS:
- **Pickled ginger, green onion, sesame seeds, wasabi, dulse flakes**

Begin by draining the package of tofu to remove excess water, then cut it lengthwise into four slices. Lay the slices flat over a couple of paper towels (or a clean kitchen towel) on top of a baking sheet. Lay a couple more paper towels over the tofu. Place another baking sheet (or heavy, flat-bottomed object) on top, plus a heavy book on top of that (because you don't want the book to get wet). Set aside for 20-30 minutes (note: you can also use a tofu press if you have one). After the tofu has been pressed, cube the tofu, transfer to a bowl and drizzle with tamari and 1 tablespoon of the rice vinegar. Set aside.

Prepare the brown rice by combining 1/2 cup brown rice with 1 cup water in a pot on the stove. Bring to a boil and cover, then reduce heat to simmer for 20 minutes, or until water is absorbed. After cooking, season the rice in the pot with a few splashes of liquid aminos and a roughly crumbled sheet of nori (or a handful of dulse flakes if you have them). Set aside.

You can cube the tofu and eat as it is or fry it in a pan with coconut oil. To fry, heat 2 teaspoons of coconut oil over medium-high heat. Once hot, add the cubed tofu and fry for five minutes on each side until lightly browned and crispy.

Before assembling the deconstructed sushi bowls, soften the kale by adding the remaining 1 tablespoon rice vinegar with the maple syrup into a bowl and massaging it into the kale leaves. Then separate the kale into two bowls, and add the tofu, brown rice and cucumber to each. Finish with the cubed avocado, extra crumbled nori and a squeeze of lemon or lime.

Note: You can also roll all ingredients into a wrap with a large nori sheet. If you prefer to steam the kale instead of eating it raw, that is fine too.

SEED CYCLING ENERGY BALLS

MAKES 10-12 BALLS

FOR OVULATORY AND LUTEAL PHASES

- 1¹/₄ cup raw sunflower seeds
- 1¹/₄ cup white sesame seeds (you can buy these online in bulk)
- ³/₄ cup vegan plant protein powder (chocolate or vanilla)
- ¹/₂ cup unsweetened shredded coconut
- ¹/₄ cup raw cacao powder (optional)
- Pinch of sea salt
- 3 tablespoons melted coconut oil
- 1–2 tablespoons maple syrup (or 10 drops stevia)
- 1 cup filtered water

Combine the sunflower seeds, sesame seeds, protein powder, coconut, cacao powder and salt in a food processor. Blend until finely ground and crumbly. Add in the coconut oil, sweetener and water, and blend until well combined and the mixture starts to form into one big ball. Using an ice cream scoop, gently form into balls (the dough is too delicate to roll). Refrigerate for 30 minutes or until firm; store in the refrigerator for snacks or to enjoy alongside your smoothies throughout the week.

FOR MENSTRUAL AND FOLLICULAR PHASES

- 1¹/₄ cup raw pumpkin seeds
- 1 ¹/₄ cup flaxseed (raw or ground)
- ³/₄ cup vegan plant protein powder (chocolate or vanilla)
- ¹/₂ cup unsweetened shredded coconut
- ¹/₄ cup raw cacao powder (optional)
- Pinch of sea salt
- 3 tablespoons melted coconut oil
- 1–2 tablespoons maple syrup (or 10 drops stevia)
- 1 cup filtered water

In a food processor, combine the pumpkin seeds, flaxseed, protein powder, coconut, cacao powder (if using) and salt. Blend until finely ground and crumbly. Add in the coconut oil, sweetener and water, and blend until well combined and the mixture begins to form into one big ball in food processor bowl. Using an ice cream scoop, gently form into balls (the dough is too delicate to roll). Refrigerate for 30 minutes or until firm; store in the refrigerator for snacks or to enjoy alongside your smoothies throughout the week.

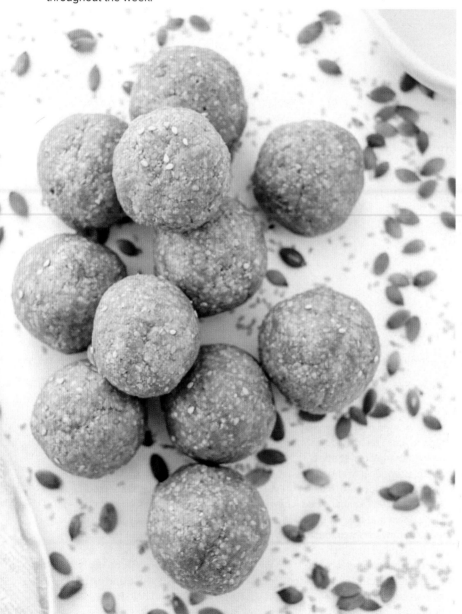

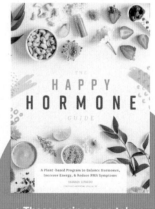

◆ These recipes are taken from Shannon Leparski's book, *The Happy Hormone Guide*, which aims to help women balance hormones and reduce PMS symptoms through a plant-based lifestyle. Discover more at **https://tinyurl.com/mwes2p69**

7 ways
to blitz your meno-middle!

Is the menopause playing havoc with your waistline? Beat belly fat, with these expert tips...

Words by Sophie Barton

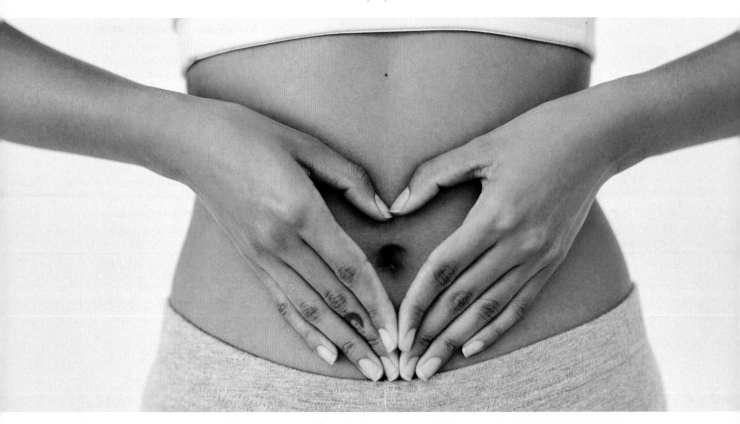

If you're having to wriggle into your jeans these days, you're not alone. Women commonly find their waistlines expanding in their 40s and 50s, due to a combination of hormonal changes and lifestyle factors. "Many women in perimenopause and early postmenopause years gain fat as their oestrogen levels drop," explains Rob Hobson, head of nutrition at Healthspan. "A change in hormone levels, mainly oestrogen, may influence body fat distribution too.

While women of childbearing age tend to store fat in the lower body, making them 'pear-shaped', postmenopausal women store fat around the abdomen, making them 'apple-shaped'. Animal studies have also shown that a lack of oestrogen leads to unwanted abdominal fat, although more research needs to be done to understand why."

But the dreaded middle-aged spread can't just be blamed on hormones, or a slowing metabolism — lifestyle factors are also often to blame. The relentless juggle of work and family responsibilities means many of us don't exercise as much as we'd like, and a sugary or stodgy diet will have an impact too. Failing to get enough shut-eye can also contribute to menopausal weight gain, as can certain medication.

Thankfully there's good news. We can blitz that belly fat, and experts Rob Hobson and Kate Rowe-Ham are here to tell you how...

1 LOOK AFTER YOUR GUT

Research suggests the menopause might affect microbiome diversity, while early animal studies suggest this change could be associated with increased body weight. So, boost your gut bacteria by eating whole foods in their most natural state. "Include fruits, veg, nuts, seeds, legumes and whole grains," adds Rob. "Include fermented foods, such as unsweetened yoghurt, kefir, kimchi, sauerkraut, and kombucha. Probiotics also supply a source of friendly bacteria (try Healthspan Super20 Pro – £17.96 for 60 capsules)."

2 OPT FOR WHOLEGRAINS

If you're suffering from 'meno-middle,' pack your diet with plenty of fibre. It helps you feel full, making it easier to regulate your appetite, plus it helps balance blood sugars, meaning less sugary cravings. It can even ease bloating and constipation. Rob recommends increasing your fibre intake by switching to wholemeal varieties of pasta and bread, and eating more wholegrains, legumes and veg.

3 QUIT CRASH DIETS

They can be tempting, but crash diets are counterproductive. "Research shows that rapid weight loss can actually reduce your metabolism," Rob explains. "That's because crash dieting triggers the body to go into survival mode, which means it burns less energy. It can also lead to nutrient insufficiencies." If you want to lose weight, take it slow and steady by eating smaller portions of nutritious food.

4 PACK IN PROTEIN

Did you know that muscle mass decreases in age, especially during menopause? Because muscle burns more energy than fat, this in turn slows the speed at which your body burns calories, making it trickier to maintain your weight. Thankfully the flip side is also true – if you preserve muscle mass, you're more likely to maintain a healthy metabolism. "This can be done through weight-bearing exercise and eating a diet rich in protein," says Rob. "Include protein, such as lean meats and oily fish, with every meal and team this with plenty of veggies and a little wholegrain carbohydrate. Protein helps support the maintenance, growth and repair of muscle tissue."

5 GET WEIGHTY

Consider swapping HIIT (high-intensity interval workouts) for some light dumbbells instead. That's because HIIT raises levels of the stress hormone cortisol. Women's health coach Kate Rowe-Ham (owningyourmenopause.com) explains, "HIIT can put us under more stress, adding to weight gain around the middle. Instead, weight training can support weight loss by burning calories during and after workouts and by preserving muscle mass, which helps prevent your metabolism from slowing. Try adding a minute of weighted squats three days a week."

6 WORK YOUR WHOLE BODY

Sit-ups might seem the obvious solution when it comes to blitzing your belly, but Kate says they won't target fat. She suggests, "Instead, add full body moves to elevate the heart rate and increase your chances of targeting fat around the middle. Go for full body moves, like mountain climbers, side planks, push-ups and squats. Do some push-ups or hold a plank whilst the kettle boils."

7 DO A DEAD BUG

Kate, founder of app, Owning Your Menopause, says it's vital to strengthen the deep muscles of your core. "A strong core can help reduce your risk of injury, as well as protecting your lower back and helping with pelvic floor issues as your oestrogen declines," she says. Kate recommends doing 'dead bugs' for a minute each morning. She explains; "Allow your shoulders and lower back to lie heavy to the floor. Draw your shoulders down away from your ears. To get into the starting position, lift your hands so your elbows are above your shoulders with your fists facing in toward each other. Lift your legs so your knees are directly over your hips. On an exhale, slowly lower your right arm and left leg until they're just above the floor. On an inhale, bring them back to the starting position. Repeat on the opposite side."

GET SOME SHUT-EYE!

Struggling to sleep? A lack of shut-eye doesn't just make you tired, it can affect your weight too. Here's why, and what you can do about it...

Have you ever noticed you crave sugary, starchy food when you're tired? Poor sleep is a common symptom of menopause, but it's also associated with weight gain and obesity too. "Sleep hygiene is the first port of call in this diet," says Rob. "Studies have suggested that people who sleep less have higher levels of ghrelin (hunger hormone) and lower levels of leptin (fullness hormone), putting them at greater risk of being overweight."

Enhance your chances of a good night's rest by going to bed and getting up at the same time each day, and consciously winding down before bedtime. That means no blue screens (leave your phone downstairs) and doing a calming activity, such as reading. If you struggle with hot flushes, try to work out if anything in particular triggers them – some people find spicy meals and hot drinks make them worse, for example.

Your diet can help in other ways too. Rob explains, "A nutritious diet will provide crucial nutrients that support the production of melatonin (sleep hormone), such as magnesium, B vitamins, and calcium. Meals rich in tryptophan, found in poultry, salmon, tofu, oats and seeds, may also help with sleep. Excess sugar can disrupt the sleep cycle too, and cutting back on stimulants such as caffeine and alcohol can also help promote sleep."

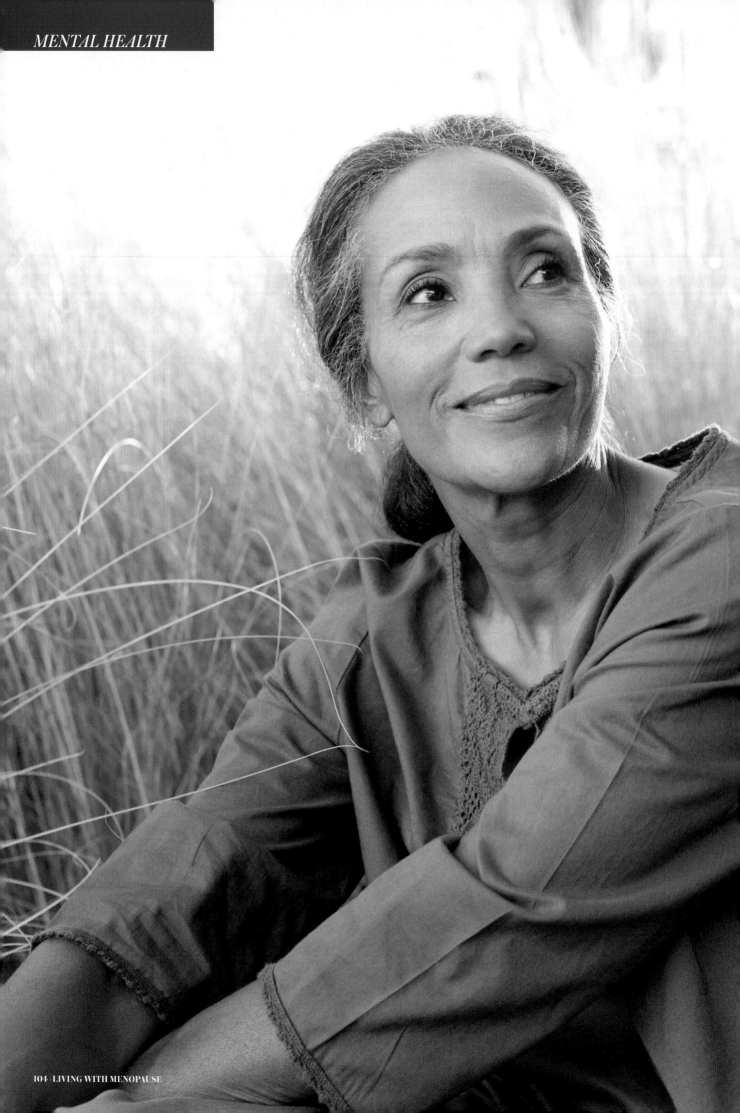

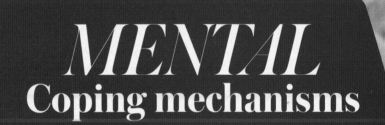

MENTAL
Coping mechanisms

It's mind over matter when dealing with menopause, as your mind really does matter

It is incredibly easy for your **mental health to take a dive while you are going through the menopause.** You become aware that you're no longer in your first youth, you go through physical changes that could be painful and your hormones go all over the place. It's perfectly normal to feel a bit down or even depressed in this situation. However, mental coping mechanisms, such as mindful practice, can help you develop a positive mindset and make sure that your frame of mind is one that will embrace the mental challenges you could face.

SURVIVING MENOPAUSE'S
Emotional Roller coaster

Why do you feel so low? Blame those raging hormones – but you can beat them

Words by Elizabeth Carr-Ellis

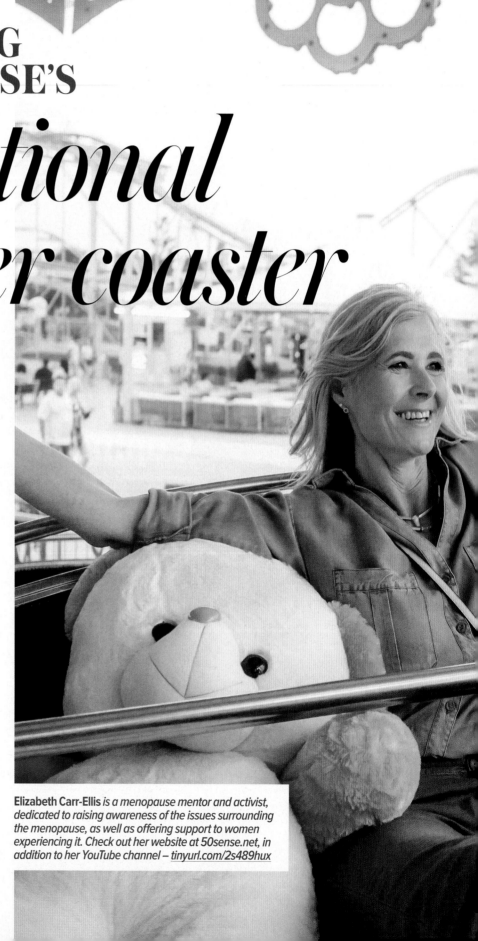

Google 'menopause' and you'll see page after page of women looking hot and sweaty, usually with a fan in their hands. But for many women, the changing hormones that come with the run-up to the menopause play a much more disruptive role on their mental health than their internal thermostat. In fact, around 70 percent of women will experience some sort of mental health issue during their menopause. For some, this can be feeling low or irritable, but others can experience much worse. Some women going through menopause will experience depression and anxiety so bad it makes them take their lives. Suicide rates have risen six percent in the last 20 years among women in the 45-54 age group – the prime age for women to go through menopause. However, while the statistics are frightening, understanding you are not alone and taking steps to counter menopausal depression and anxiety can help get you through.

Elizabeth Carr-Ellis *is a menopause mentor and activist, dedicated to raising awareness of the issues surrounding the menopause, as well as offering support to women experiencing it. Check out her website at 50sense.net, in addition to her YouTube channel – tinyurl.com/2s489hux*

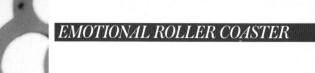

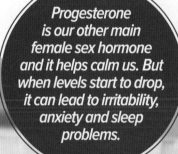

> Progesterone is our other main female sex hormone and it helps calm us. But when levels start to drop, it can lead to irritability, anxiety and sleep problems.

GET BACK THE LOVING FEELING

Divorce rates for women peak in their 40s – the prime time for perimenopause. Low hormone levels can leave many women feeling irritable and angry over the slightest thing, leading to arguments with their family, partner or work colleagues. Some women, however, will instead try to suppress their emotions and stay quiet, fuelling their own feelings of inadequacy and resentment. In addition, the fall in testosterone can leave women with a low sex drive and while they may still love their partner, they no longer feel the impetus to make love. Good communication is key to surviving the emotional maelstrom, together with finding new ways to add intimacy to your relationship, such as non-penetrative sex or a simple cuddle in bed. And at a time when physical and emotional symptoms can impact on how a woman feels about her body, self-care becomes crucial to relieve the stress and strains.

CULTURAL IMPACT

Every woman experiences their own menopause, with different symptoms and feelings. However, cultural differences can play a major part in how symptoms will hit, with studies showing that women from different ethnic backgrounds display different symptoms or experience them to a stronger or lesser extent. Women living in cultures where older women are revered and menopause is seen as a time of positive change often experience few and less debilitating symptoms. In those cultures that see ageing as negative and view menopause as a time of lowering sexual allure, women suffer more. Coming at a time when women often feel their confidence and self-esteem hit by changing hormones, such negative messages have been found to have a negative impact on their mental health, leaving them prone to depression and anxiety. It can also make women feel ashamed of being menopausal, leading them to delay seeking help.

Getting through the change

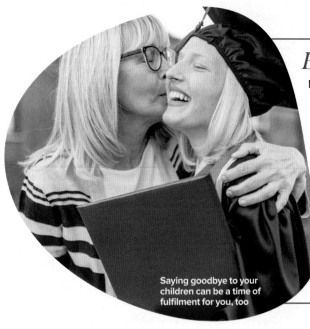

Saying goodbye to your children can be a time of fulfilment for you, too

EMPTY NEST SYNDROME

Many parents find themselves at a loss when their children leave the home, either for work or university, but it can hit menopausal women particularly hard. Suddenly feeling unwanted after 18 or so years supplying all of their child's needs leaves a lot of women feeling their purpose in life has gone. This can be particularly challenging for women already in a more fragile state with their changing hormones, causing them to feel lonely and lost. Ironically, for some, the conflicting emotions may leave them craving a new baby to fill the hole. Despite this, many women find that once they get used to the change, they can start to focus on their own wants and needs for the first time. Some return to further education or find a new challenge at work, even starting their own business. It is an opportunity to find the real you!

AGEING PARENTS

While their children may be leaving the nest, many menopausal women find they suddenly have someone else to care for – their parents. Menopause often collides with the time our parents or older relatives start losing their health, either physically or mentally. Caring for an ailing parent can exacerbate menopause symptoms and impact both the caregiver's health and their ability to look after their loved one. In addition, they may also have to juggle the needs of their parents with the needs of their own children, helping out with grandchildren, for example, and feel pulled in different directions. Support networks are a great way to get through this time, with many women finding relief by talking through their feelings with friends and other relatives, while there are many online groups available. See if there is a local Menopause Café you can attend, to meet others in similar situations (menopausecafe.net).

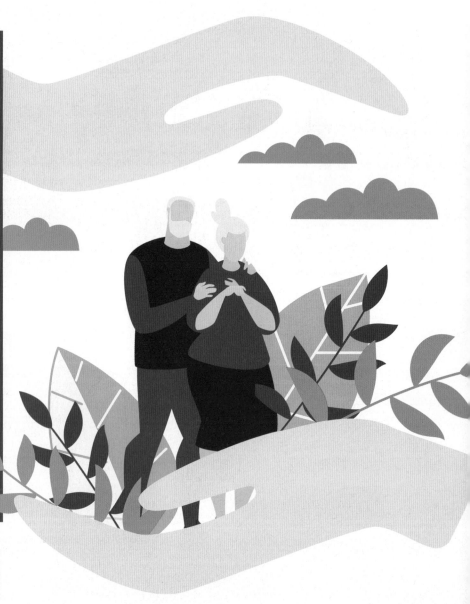

It can be difficult suddenly finding yourself having to care for the person who cared for you

EMBRACE THE CHANGE

After the confidence and strength of our youth, menopause can be a wake-up call that we are not, after all, immortal. In the years leading up to the menopause itself – that magic moment when we are 12 months without a period – it can feel as if life is nothing but decay. But once through, many women find they feel a new sense of freedom, and they are renewed – echoing the Chinese view that menopause is a 'second spring'. PMS and inconvenient periods in the middle of a holiday are things of the past, as is the fear of becoming pregnant. With the lowering of hormones comes the lowering of hormonal problems, such as a reduction in migraines and other headaches. Most importantly, it is a time to take stock and take a fresh look at your life. Yes, it is 'the change' – but how that change goes is up to you.

Be the change – enjoy your postmenopause life

Oestrogen impacts your serotonin – your happy hormone. When it starts declining, so does your serotonin, which is why you can feel more tearful or even depressed.

You may need extra help to remember vital things

CUT THROUGH THE FOG

Oestrogen doesn't just affect our serotonin, it also plays a huge part in our cognitive functions. As a result, it's common for women to become more forgetful or suffer from brain fog or brain fatigue. Many also find their concentration levels are not as strong as they were, while everyday tasks can seem like an uphill struggle. Women can feel frustrated both at themselves and others. In addition, sleep can become a problem, with women either struggling to fall asleep or waking several times a night, and this adds to the difficulties they experience through the day. Techniques such as meditation and mindfulness can help cut through the fog and focus the mind, together with good sleep hygiene, such as going to bed at a regular time and stopping the use of smartphones or computer screens for an hour before bed.

MENOPAUSE AND
depression

How to recognise the signs of depression during menopause and tips on how to beat it

Words by Suzy Stanton

Menopause can be **accompanied by many symptoms, from restless legs to brain fog, hot flushes, anxiety, and depression.** Many women go through this phase of their life without experiencing any of those symptoms. But for some, they can have a massive impact on how they live.

Depression is one of the symptoms that can have the biggest impact on a woman's life, particularly if they've experienced it in the past. Symptoms are usually at their most severe at certain points of the menstrual cycle, which can have a profound impact on those affected. It's therefore important to know how to recognise the signs and have strategies in place to manage the symptoms.

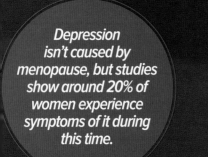

Depression isn't caused by menopause, but studies show around 20% of women experience symptoms of it during this time.

TOP TIPS FOR MANAGING DEPRESSION

Knowing your triggers can help you manage symptoms so they don't take over your life.

Depression that is connected to menopause tends to be cyclical. Monitoring your symptoms over a few months will help you work out when it's likely to be worse. You can then put together a tool kit of things that help during those times. Here are some strategies that may help:

EXERCISE

Exercise, or even just moving your body more energetically than you normally would, releases feel-good brain chemicals like endorphins that can enhance your sense of well-being and lift your mood. You don't have to run a marathon or do an hour-long HIIT class to get the benefit. Do what you enjoy, whether that's a brisk walk in your local park or dancing to some favourite tunes around your kitchen.

As little as 15 minutes of exercise can make a difference to feelings of low mood and depression; 30 minutes three times a week can have a significant impact.

EAT A HEALTHY DIET

Eating a healthy diet doesn't mean restricting what you eat. It means having a good balance. So, plenty of fruit and vegetables, healthy protein, carbohydrates, with the odd pudding and treat too. Cooking from scratch is the best way of making sure what you eat is balanced. Again, it doesn't have to be complicated. Using a slow cooker is a great way of creating healthy meals, easily, and is cheaper to use than a conventional oven, so it's helping your pocket too.

WRITE THINGS DOWN

If you're feeling low or anxious, writing down how you feel can help you manage your thoughts. It helps you see whether your worries are something you can control and if they are, put a plan together to tackle the problem. If it's something you can't control, try and let it go.

BE MINDFUL

Mindfulness is a powerful tool to manage depression and anxiety. Being more aware of what we're doing and our thoughts and feelings, helps us notice when we're feeling down. Noticing feelings can help you distance yourself from them.

Mindfulness doesn't have to be complicated. Some people find meditation helps them manage their feelings better. For others, it can be as simple as having a few moments alone, taking some deep breaths, and noticing their feelings.

MAKE A MENTAL HEALTH FIRST AID KIT

Having some go-to activities that help you when you're feeling down, can help you manage depression symptoms effectively. We all have some kind of physical first aid kit, even if it's just a couple of paracetamol and plasters. But having a mental health first aid kit is just as important. It can be physical – perhaps a box of things that help like a colouring book and pens, chocolate or a book. Or it can be a note in your phone or notebook, of all the things that help you feel better when your mood is low.

MEDICATION

If your symptoms are severe, talk to your GP about medication, such as HRT and antidepressants.

"Exercise releases feel-good brain chemicals that can lift your mood"

THE MAIN SYMPTOMS OF DEPRESSION

Symptoms vary for each person – here are some of the most common ones to look out for:

- Feeling down or upset and tearful. Your get up and go feels like it has got up and left.
- Agitated, on edge, irritable and restless. Snapping at those around you and generally acting out of character.
- Brain fog – finding it difficult to concentrate, think clearly or make decisions. This makes work difficult.
- Feeling worthless and down on yourself. Hiding away and avoiding the activities you usually enjoy.
- Losing your confidence and self-esteem, feeling isolated and unable to relate to people.
- Feeling hopeless.
- Difficulty sleeping or sleeping too much. Feeling tired all the time regardless of how much sleep you've had.
- Losing interest in sex.
- Change in appetite.
- Aches and pains with no obvious physical reason.
- Losing interest in your appearance.

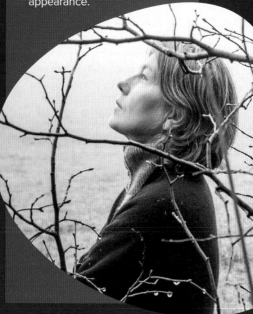

COPING WITH *Brain Fog*

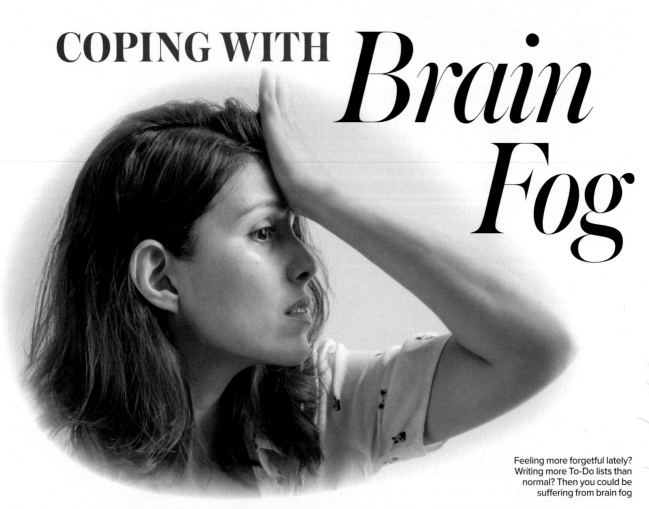

Feeling more forgetful lately? Writing more To-Do lists than normal? Then you could be suffering from brain fog

Once like a sponge, now like cotton wool, your brain feels like it's changing too...

Words by Natalie Denton

Brain fog – the cloudy feeling that seems to make remembering and retaining information more difficult than before – is said to affect around two-thirds of menopausal and perimenopausal women.

If you feel you're becoming increasingly forgetful, maybe forgetting why you walked in a room, or finding it harder to retain information, follow a conversation or stay focused, you could be suffering from brain fog. The good news is most women recover after going through the change, but there are some things that can help in the meantime. Here's the lowdown on what's actually happening and what you can do to cope.

FIND A BALANCE

It's thought declining levels of progesterone and oestrogen are the main culprits behind menopausal-related memory loss because among other things, they aid concentration span, language skills, mood and memory. One way to tackle the effects of brain fog is by dealing with the imbalance of hormones. This includes adopting a healthy lifestyle, de-stressing and brain-training exercises to improve cognitive function.

GET SOME REST

Another contributing factor of brain fog is the lack of sleep women typically endure during the change, so anything you do to get a good night's sleep will help. Avoid eating a heavy meal or drinking caffeine before bed and relax with breathing exercises or meditation.

CHECK YOUR BLOOD PRESSURE

Women with hypertension (high blood pressure) are said to have a 30 percent increased risk of developing cognitive impairment, so book yourself in for a health check with your GP and have your blood pressure examined. If it's very high they can prescribe medication to bring it down, or suggest some natural and herbal alternatives.

GET MOVING

Regular aerobic exercise and strength training provide a bounty of benefits for the body and mind. In relation to brain fog, exercise improves blood flow to the brain ensuring it's working at its best, and as with all physical activity, will provide a rush of endorphins that'll boost your mood and improve your quality of sleep.

YOU ARE WHAT YOU EAT

Look after your diet and your diet will look after you. Forgo processed and fatty foods (particularly trans fats), diet drinks, cigarettes, and limit your intake of alcohol. Instead pursue whole foods, fruit and vegetables in order to feed your brain with all the vitamins and minerals it needs.

CHANGING YOUR MENOPAUSE
Mindset

Don't accept that the menopause will be hell – take steps to embrace a positive outlook and turn it into a life event where you thrive, rather then just survive

Words by Jo Cole

KNOWLEDGE IS POWER

A big old research session into what happens during the menopause, what causes the symptoms and what can help lessen them (diet, vitamins, etc), is very empowering. Okay, so it won't stop you experiencing symptoms, but understanding why something is happening reduces anxiety and makes it easier to stay positive..

STOP PLAYING THE SHAME GAME

Do you tell yourself to stop being so silly when your hormones are playing havoc with your mood and body? You don't need to do this. Take some deep breaths, accept what is happening and know that it will pass. Making peace with the bad times frees you up for good times!

KEEP A JOURNAL

A journal is an excellent way of organising the maelstrom of thoughts churning in your mind, as well as being somewhere you can vent your feelings, instead of keeping them bottled up. Plus, the process of sitting and writing can be calming, leaving you relaxed and ready for the world.

CATCH UP WITH FRIENDS

Having a good laugh about the menopause with friends is one of the most positive activites you can do. Not only will this improve your mood, but instead of feeling down the next time you have a menopause-related incident, think about how you will tell the story to the gang.

REFLECT ON THE PAST

There is a stigma attached to the menopause that it is the final chapter of a woman's life. Forget that way of thinking; see the menopause as a time to reflect upon what you have achieved and experienced. Feel proud of where you are and what you've learnt and be excited for what comes next.

LOOK TO THE FUTURE

One symptom of the menopause – the reduced ability to gloss over irritations in your life – can be harnessed for good. Without oestrogen supplying rose-tinted glasses for the parts of your life that annoy you, take an honest assessment of what you don't like and then do something about it. Be liberated by the menopause!

GET FIGHTING FIT

Having a fitness regime during the menopause not only improves mood, but will stop you losing muscle mass, reduce the risk of heart disease and cancer, improve your skin and keep your bones strong. Strength training is one of the best forms of exercise for this stage of life, so get to it!

WELCOME DISTRACTIONS

It's hard to remain positive when you are being hammered by hormonal hurricanes, so set yourself up with a pile of distractions to turn to if you're heading for a negative spiral. Books, hobbies, podcasts, music, TV or films... anything that you can concentrate on to replace discomfort with joy.

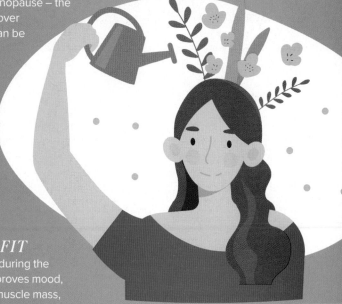

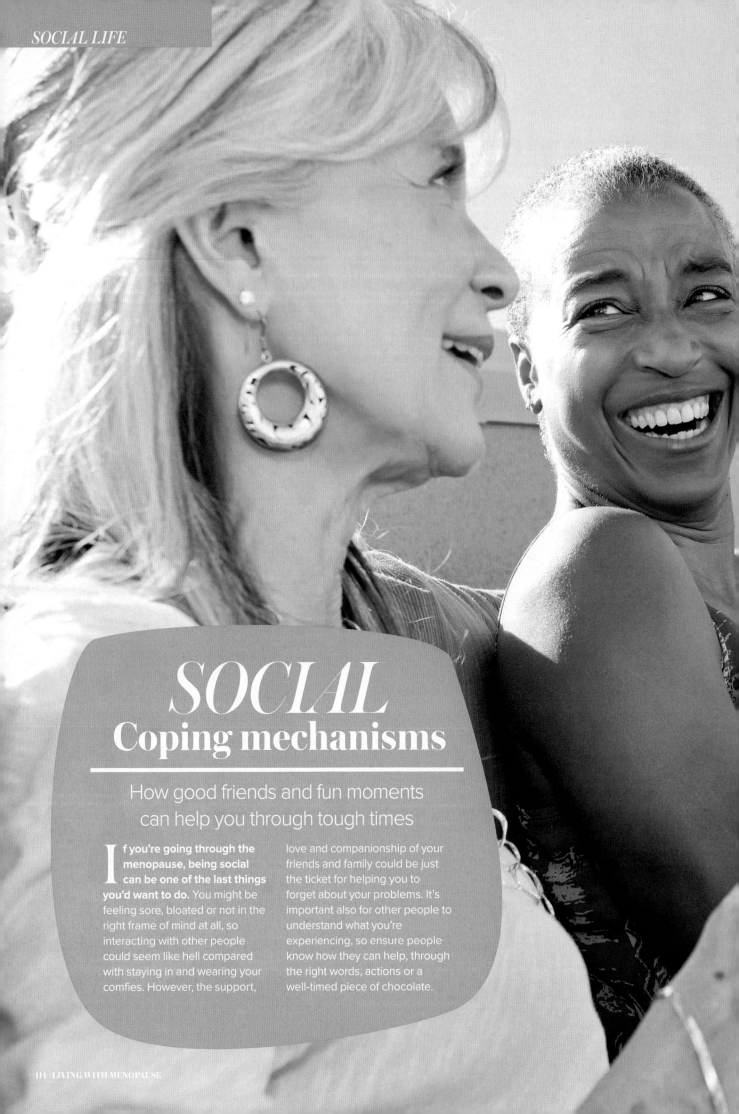

SOCIAL
Coping mechanisms

How good friends and fun moments can help you through tough times

If you're going through the **menopause, being social can be one of the last things you'd want to do.** You might be feeling sore, bloated or not in the right frame of mind at all, so interacting with other people could seem like hell compared with staying in and wearing your comfies. However, the support, love and companionship of your friends and family could be just the ticket for helping you to forget about your problems. It's important also for other people to understand what you're experiencing, so ensure people know how they can help, through the right words, actions or a well-timed piece of chocolate.

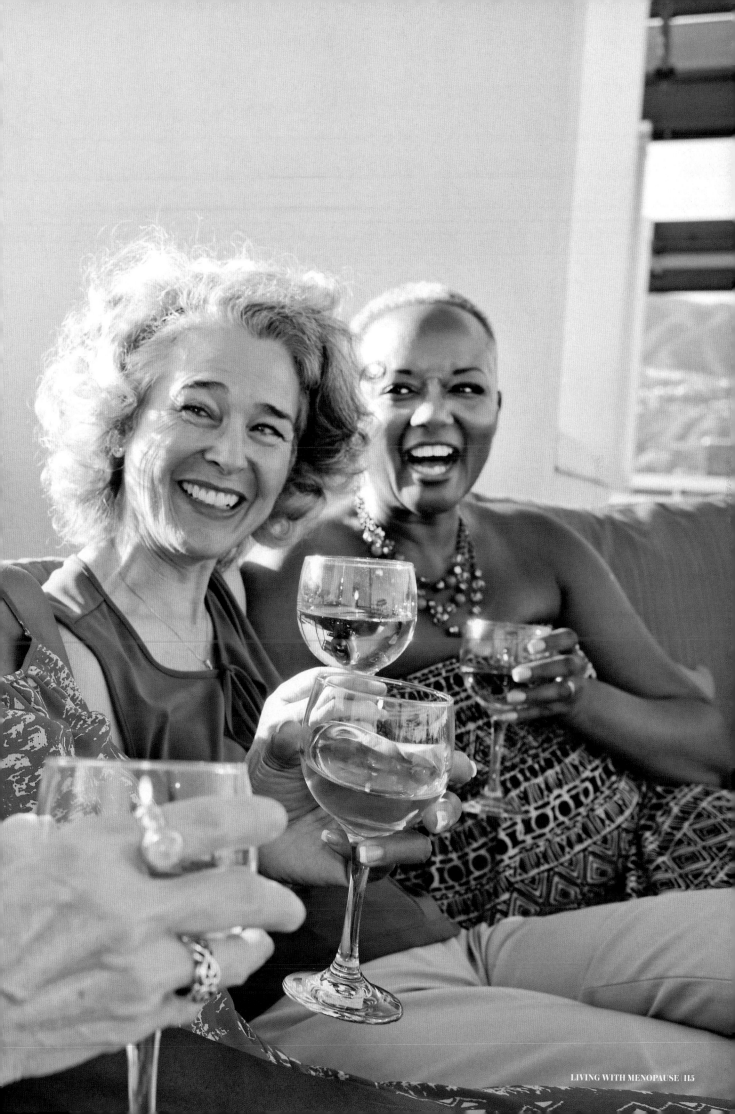

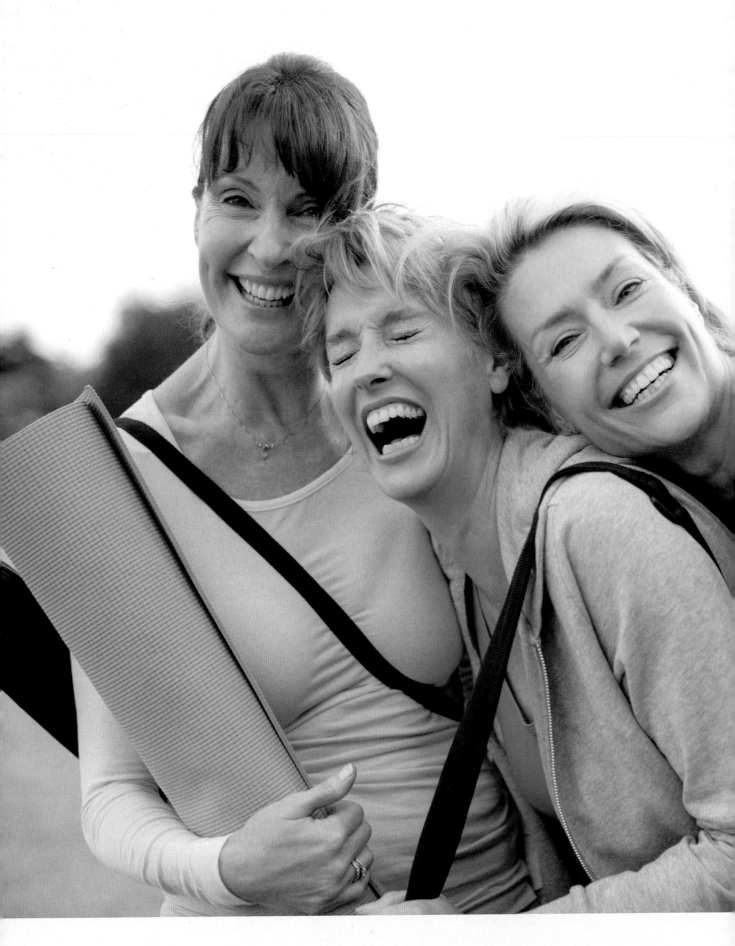

GETTING SUPPORT

Whether it's tackling hot flushes or feeling like you're on an emotional rollercoaster, you don't need to do menopause alone

Words by Jenna Farmer

Menopause, the time in our lives when our menstrual cycles come to an end, used to be a taboo topic. Feeling as if they had no choice but to keep quiet, millions of women in their 40s and 50s had to struggle through 'the change' without accessing the support they really needed. Thankfully, advocates such as Davina McCall, have paved the way for us to now talk openly about menopause – something that 13 million women in the UK are currently going through. It's a huge number and a reminder you're not alone during the menopause, even if it can sometimes feel that way.

Of course, some women breeze through this time in their lives but for others, it's more challenging: 77 percent of women have at least one menopause symptom they have difficulty dealing with, but many are still reluctant to chat openly with their GP. However, the menopause is a normal stage of your life and nothing to be embarrassed about. Getting support from those around you (such as your GP, loved ones and boss) is key to helping you thrive during it. So how can you ensure you have the support to embrace this part of your life and deal with the challenges it may bring? Read on for our top tips...

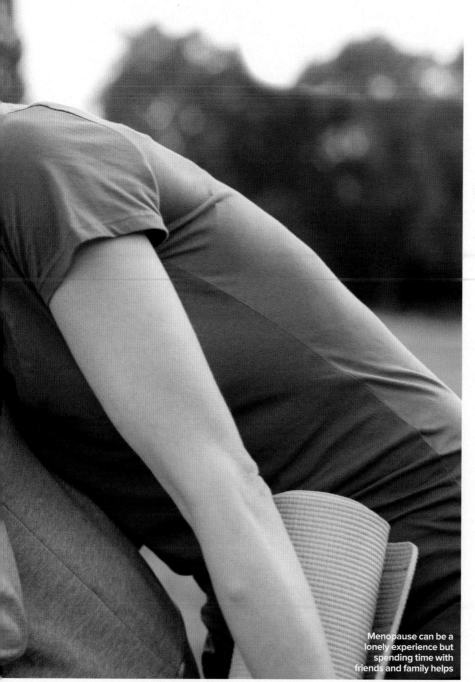

Menopause can be a lonely experience but spending time with friends and family helps

HOW TO SUPPORT YOURSELF

Menopause can impact the most important relationship in your life — the one with yourself

Although you need support from others during menopause, it's also important to work on your relationship with yourself. Some women internalise the embarrassment they feel about menopause and turn it into self-doubt and negative thinking. Sound familiar? Well firstly, being more open about what you're going through will make a real difference to the type of support you can receive. If you don't yet feel confident enough to broach the subject with others in your life, why not join an online menopause support group to make connections? Maybe use Instagram to find accounts of others going through menopause.

Menopause can impact things like your confidence, self-esteem and body image; whether that's due to mood changes (perimenopausal women can be at risk of depression in particular) or body changes. For example, lower levels of oestrogen can lead to issues like drier skin and increased hair loss, or women may notice weight fluctuations. If you can afford it, investing in skincare and haircare products to adapt to these changes could help. Take time when you get dressed each morning to appreciate your new body — you could try repeating a self-confidence mantra (such as "my body is changing and I am okay with that") as you do.

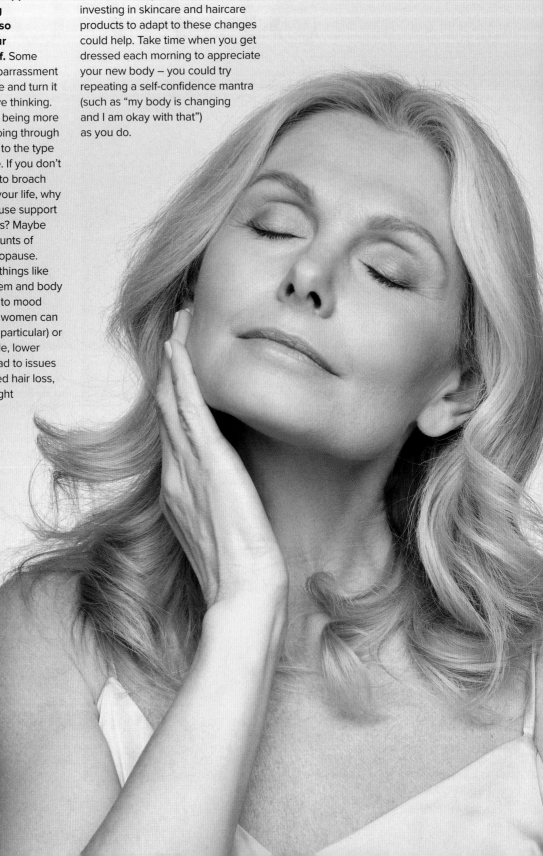

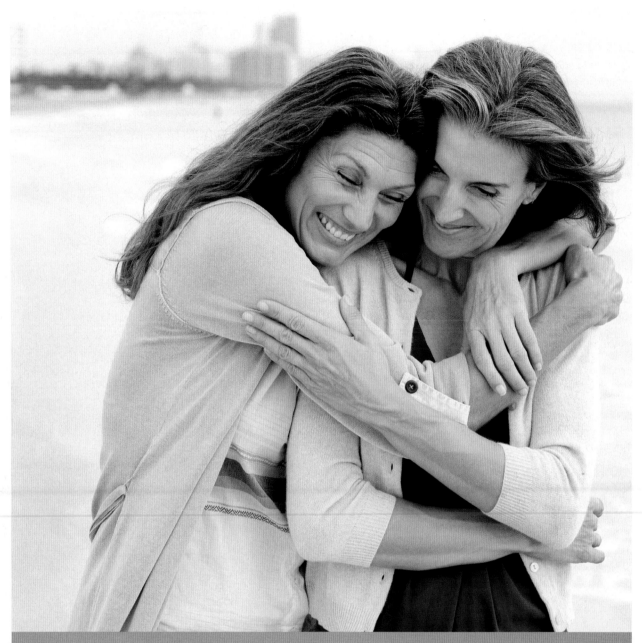

HOW TO GET SUPPORT FROM FAMILY AND FRIENDS

Menopause expert Meera Bhogal shares her top tips to feeling supported through menopause with the help of loved ones

Feeling lonely during menopause is common, but speaking to family and friends can really help. "Menopause can be a lonely journey and one which is riddled with anxiety and fear of the unknown," explains menopause expert Meera Bhogal. "Sharing your journey with those who love you can make a huge difference to how you experience this stage of your life," she adds.

So how can we build these relationships? "Share with them the

factual information so they also understand that this is a natural stage of every woman's life and what the symptoms may be," says Meera. For many, lack of support could simply be due to not understanding menopause, so stick to the facts when explaining what it is like.

But is there anything that can be done when you are dealing with menopausal mood swings, which impact over 20 percent of women? "Ask family and friends to give you

space and time – but also be honest when you're being irrational. Sometimes menopause can make us feel like we don't want to do simple things that can help – like meeting friends. Family and friends can gently help us unpick this (without ridiculing of course) to help us rationalise again," Meera adds.

♦ **Meera is the founder of the Don't Pause for Menopause programme, meerabhogal.com**

HOW TO GET SUPPORT FROM YOUR WORKPLACE

Many menopausal women work, but many workplaces need to do more to help their staff going through menopause

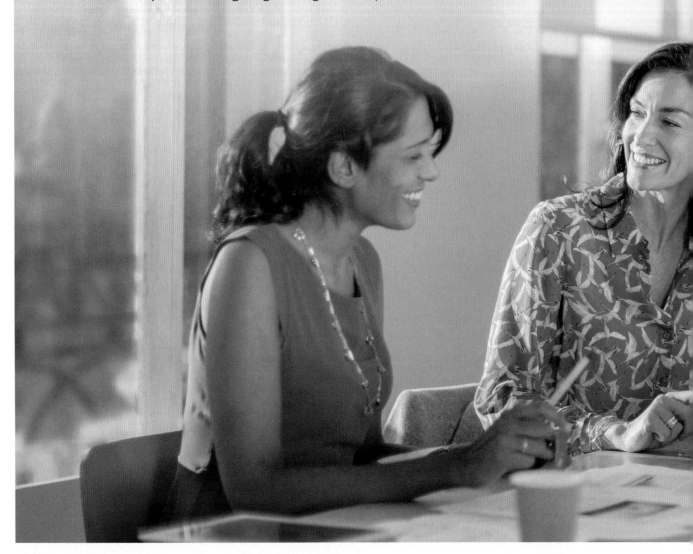

Menopausal women make up a huge part of our workforce – in fact, they're the fastest growing demographic in the workplace. There's no reason why you can't have the career of your dreams in your 40s, 50s (and beyond), but having support is key. Research has found that a quarter of women have actually considered leaving their job because of menopause.

Remember, you have the right to ask for any reasonable adjustments that would make your working life easier and to do the amazing work you know you're capable of. Before you approach your employer, think about what could be done to help you manage. This will vary depending on your symptoms and the type of work you do but flexible working is a great place to start. If you are dealing with hot flushes, asking for flexibility in the uniform you wear (Nottinghamshire Police were the first force in the UK to implement lighter-weight police

uniforms) or even being able to use air con can feel like a life-saver.

Many menopausal women struggle from brain fog, which can be frustrating when you're used to managing big projects. However, ask to use software that enables you to set reminders or take notes, or for more regular breaks to give your brain a chance to recharge. Either way, it's important to be open with HR about how menopause is impacting you and what they can do to meet your needs.

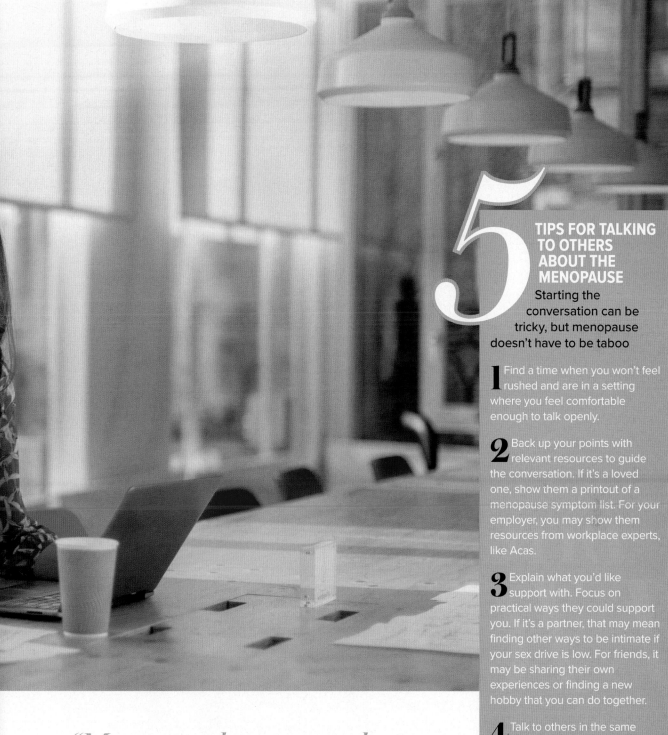

5 TIPS FOR TALKING TO OTHERS ABOUT THE MENOPAUSE

Starting the conversation can be tricky, but menopause doesn't have to be taboo

1 Find a time when you won't feel rushed and are in a setting where you feel comfortable enough to talk openly.

2 Back up your points with relevant resources to guide the conversation. If it's a loved one, show them a printout of a menopause symptom list. For your employer, you may show them resources from workplace experts, like Acas.

3 Explain what you'd like support with. Focus on practical ways they could support you. If it's a partner, that may mean finding other ways to be intimate if your sex drive is low. For friends, it may be sharing their own experiences or finding a new hobby that you can do together.

4 Talk to others in the same boat. You might join a local menopause coffee morning, or find an online support group if you would prefer not to do things face-to-face.

5 Take notes. This is really important if you're talking to your doctor. Go armed with a list of your symptoms and any questions you may have.

"Menopausal women make up a huge part of our workforce – in fact, they're actually the fastest growing demographic in the workplace"

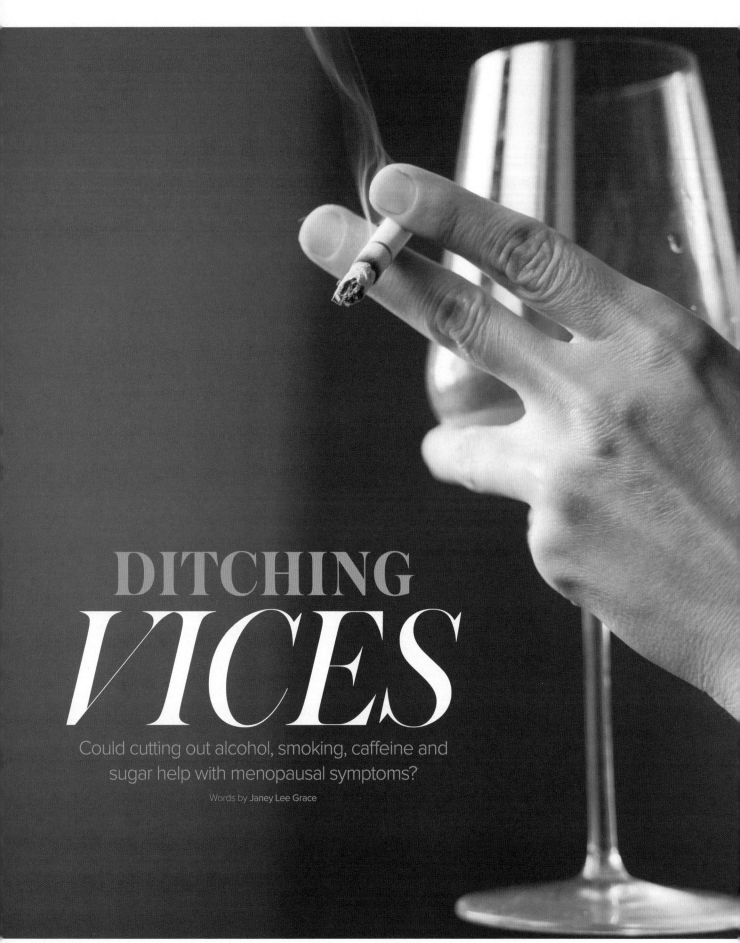

DITCHING
VICES

Could cutting out alcohol, smoking, caffeine and
sugar help with menopausal symptoms?

Words by Janey Lee Grace

Although you are unable to avoid the menopause, there is actually quite a lot you can do to try and mitigate the symptoms. That's the good news. The bad news is that the easiest place to start is also the hardest to implement – taking a look at your lifestyle and dealing with the areas that make menopausal symptoms worse. Alcohol, smoking, caffeine and sugar can all increase the severity of symptoms, which of course ironically, are the very vices you might turn to when you are feeling rubbish. It's therefore important to understand how each one affects common symptoms, so you are able to make informed choices about what you can change to make life that little bit easier.

ALCOHOL AND THE MENOPAUSE

Drinking for pleasure, or social drinking, can bring enjoyment with friends and family, help you celebrate a special occasion or unwind after a hard day. However, it can also exacerbate menopausal symptoms. Women tend to be more vulnerable to the effects of alcohol, partly because the enzyme that metabolises it, dehydrogenase, is fairly inactive in our liver, so we absorb more alcohol in our bloodstream. Also as we age, our tendons and cartilage lose water, which means our body holds less water. The more water in your body, the better you can dilute alcohol.

Studies have shown that alcohol can disrupt sleep, as well as make hot flushes and night sweats worse. However, there are other studies that assert alcohol can actually help with hot flushes. Women who drink once a month appear less likely to have hot flushes than women who drink no alcohol. The severity of the flushes are also less. Talk about mixed messages! The key here is frequency. A drink now and then probably won't have you breaking out in the mother of all hot flushes, but drinking regularly might.

The North American Menopause Society states that a woman who drinks between two and five glasses of alcohol a day during menopause will

If you find it difficult to give up a vice, make sure you get help. Either visit your doctor for advice, or search online for support groups in your area. You don't have to go through anything alone.

"Alcohol can disrupt sleep and make hot flushes worse"

increase the risk of cancer, heart disease and osteoporoses. The hormonal havoc caused by the menopause already increases the risk of these, so excess alcohol makes this even worse. This is also the case with depression – both menopause and alcohol can cause depression, so when you put the two together, the risk becomes greater.

It's also easy to forget that alcohol contains a lot of sugar, so can disrupt blood sugar levels. You should aim for stable levels during menopause, as this helps keep your moods balanced.

We all know that excessive alcohol consumption is bad for us – menopause or not – but if you like your wine or beer, the occasional drink won't hurt. However, if you find your symptoms get worse after drinking, it might be time to stop!

WHY NOW IS THE TIME TO QUIT SMOKING

We all know the dangers of smoking, but if you are a smoker and have never quite managed to quit, the effect it has on menopausal symptoms might be enough to persuade you.

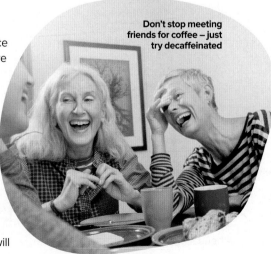

Don't stop meeting friends for coffee – just try decaffeinated

"Because of the declining levels of oestrogen, your sensitivity to insulin is reduced"

For starters, there is evidence that smoking increases your risk of early menopause. This can not only play havoc with fertility, but brings a raft of other health issues. Early menopause increases the risk of type 2 diabetes, heart disease and osteoporosis. The chances of suffering from depression and anxiety are also higher.

Smoking gives your nervous system a kick up the butt, which can make you feel as though you have more energy. This is the ideal launchpad for hot flushes. A nervous system that is firing on all cylinders can also cause or increase feelings of anxiety or contribute to mood swings.

The declining hormones in a menopausal body can play havoc with skin, causing it to feel dry and papery. Smoking also affects skin in this way, so when the two combine, you can end up with skin that feels like parchment.

And there's more. Smoking can cause larger stomachs, less muscle mass and decreased bone density. And as you will know by now from this publication, all of those are side effects of the menopause, so it's just another example of a bad situation being made worse by smoking.

Given all of the evidence, if ever there was a time to quit, the menopause is surely it.

CAFFEINE BLUES

It can seem as though everywhere you look, people are walking about with their takeaway cups of drink, as if it's unthinkable to be away from a caffeine source for any period of time. Meeting up for a coffee or cup of tea is also an excuse to take a break or meet up with friends and colleagues.

And while we would never wish to take someone's caffeine away from them, the effect it can have on menopausal symptoms is worth knowing. Drink a lot of caffeine and you could be looking at increased hot flushes and night sweats. A study by the Mayo Clinic found this seemed to be the case in postmenopausal women, however in perimenopausal women, caffeine appeared to help with mood, memory and concentration.

Caffeine can also contribute to palpitations, trouble sleeping and headaches. All three of these become more common during the menopause, so if you find you suffer from any of these symptoms, consider reducing your caffeine intake to see if it helps.

NOT SO SWEET

Sugar – that source of so much dopamine-induced joy – also has a part to play in the intensity of menopause symptoms. If your blood is full of glucose your body produces more the stress hormone, cortisol. Increased levels of cortisol interferes with hormone balance because it squashes how much progesterone can be produced. The result of this? Your periods will be irregular and most likely heavier, plus you might feel more anxious, depressed and suffer from hot flushes more often.

Cortisol is produced by the adrenal glands, which also start producing oestrogen when the ovaries wind down. If they are being forced to produce more cortisol, they won't be producing oestrogen. Your body reacts to this by storing fat around the tummy, and using this to produce oestrogen. A clever move, no doubt, but it does increase the risk of heart disease.

But this increased cortisol/declining oestrogen pattern has another consequence. It can affect how well the thyroid functions, which sets up how fast your metabolism is and how much energy you have.

Also, because of the declining levels of oestrogen during menopause, your sensitivity to insulin is reduced. This means that your ability to rid the blood of sugar is hampered, therefore raising the risk of type 2 diabetes.

And there's more. One symptom of the menopause is an increased risk of urinary tract infections (UTIs) and thrush. If you consume a lot of sugar, you are feeding the unhelpful bacteria in your body, which you guessed it, can go on to cause UTIs and thrush.

WHAT NOW?

If you decide to drastically cut your consumption of a vice – or maybe give it up – don't focus on what you're giving up, but what you are gaining. Avoiding detrimental symptoms can be a great incentive to finally cut down on things you know are doing you harm.

Make sure you have something to replace the vice. When you aren't reaching for a drink or a sugary snack you may find you have extra time. Use this to focus on self-care, perhaps revisit a hobby you used to enjoy.

It's also important to focus on good nutrition, at least for the first six weeks of ditching a vice. This is not the time to be dieting or fasting! Ideally have three meals a day and protein with every meal. This will help balance the brain chemistry. Eat foods that support the menopause – you can find lots of information in this publication about what to chomp down on.

Of course, you might find that your usual vices play no part in making symptoms worse – every woman experiences a different menopause. However, by understanding how alcohol, smoking, caffeine and sugar can affect your body during menopause, you have a few more tricks up your sleeve when it comes to showing your symptoms who is boss!

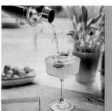

KEEP THE RITUAL, CHANGE THE INGREDIENTS
Fortunately you don't need to feel left out if you are cutting back on alcohol or caffeine. There is now a huge choice of excellent low- and no-alcohol drinks – everything from alcohol-free beer and spirits, through to artisan tonics. Or try a herbal tea for a hot drink fix.

The Guys' Guide
TO THE MENOPAUSE

There isn't a lot of guidance or literature for the male partners of women experiencing menopause, so we're here to cover the basics

1 START AT THE BEGINNING
If you find yourself at a loss with how to help the menopausal woman in your life, the best place to start is making sure you really understand what the menopause is and how it might affect your partner. Take the time to familiarise yourself with educational material.

2 BE SUPPORTIVE
If your partner is amenable to the idea, offer to keep her company at meetings with doctors and medical professionals. You'll find yourself absorbing a lot of information (with the added bonus of providing your loved one with emotional and practical support).

3 BE PATIENT
Symptoms of the menopause can last for varying amounts of time – from a few months to a few years. It's important you accept that your partner could be affected for a significant amount of time before she will feel 'herself' again.

4 TALK ABOUT IT
Open communication is vital to every healthy relationship – and especially so during the time of perimenopause and menopause. Make sure your partner knows that you want to be helpful in any way you can be, and that you want to understand how she might be feeling and what she might be thinking.

5 IT'S NOT ABOUT YOU
Your partner may be feeling distressed, anxious, depressed, or lacking in confidence during her menopause, and sometimes these mood swings might feel directed at you. Remember not to take anything personally as they are not a reflection on you – she's just experiencing a challenging time.

6 ADAPT TO CHANGES IN YOUR SEX LIFE
Your partner's body is changing, as well as her sex drive and attitude to sex. Her libido may be low, but will likely revive after the menopause, so don't be pushy. If your partner is experiencing pain, encourage her to talk to a doctor for solutions instead of suffering in silence.

"Don't take anything personally"

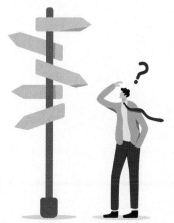

Being in an intimate relationship with a woman going through the menopause can be a new and confusing experience for men

7 KEEP ROMANCE ALIVE
If sexual intimacy between you and your partner is not what it once was, remember that you can still be intimate in other ways. Make sure your partner knows that she's still beautiful to you and that you keep the fires of passion stoked with romantic dates.

8 SUPPORT HER DIET AND EXERCISE CHANGES
Menopausal women may find that dietary changes can help relieve symptoms associated with menopause, while physical fitness can help maintain muscle strength, manage weight gain, and provide an outlet for stress. Why not join in and maybe see an improvement in your own health at the same time?

9 VALIDATE HER SYMPTOMS AND FEELINGS
Entering perimenopause is a slow transition and there's no test that can confirm it has 'officially' started. If your partner feels different and believes that she has started feeling symptoms, be compassionate and supportive and validate her feelings instead of doubting her.

10 FIND HELP IF YOU NEED IT
If you find yourself feeling negatively affected by your partner's emotions or are struggling to cope, you may also benefit from some professional help. Ask a doctor or therapist, or approach a trusted friend if you need some support during this unpredictable time.

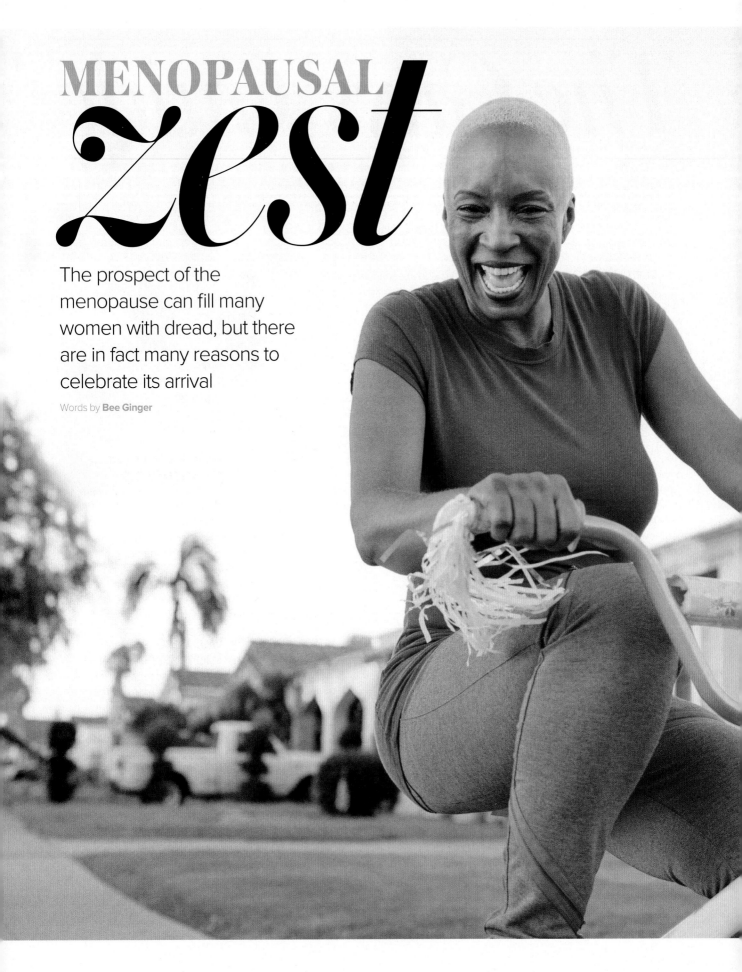

MENOPAUSAL
Zest

The prospect of the menopause can fill many women with dread, but there are in fact many reasons to celebrate its arrival

Words by **Bee Ginger**

W hen we think of the menopause, the images we conjure up in our heads may not always be positive. The list of unwelcome symptoms can often be a little daunting, not to mention disheartening, but in fact there are also many positives to be found as you embark on this next stage of your life. Here we learn a little about how in many ways, the menopause may end up being a welcome change.

SAY GOODBYE TO PERIODS!

The end of the menstrual cycle is a huge cause for celebration for many women. The guessing game of the perimenopause and its irregular periods are gone, as is the need for pads, tampons and worries about leakage, plus menstrual cramping is a thing of the past. For many who have suffered heavy bleeding, the end of periods can be fantastically liberating.

SHOCK-FREE SEX

Reports show that many women who reach menopause find they enjoy sex more as they no longer have to worry about unplanned pregnancies.

LUNCH, LAUGH, SHARE

Bonding with other women over menopause experiences can help to create a kinship. By talking things over and joking about symptoms, you will feel assured that you are not on your own. You might even learn some new coping methods. Be assured that it really won't last forever.

CHEERIO FIBROIDS!

Fibroids develop in the body when oestrogen levels are high – for example during pregnancy and in perimenopause, when levels have taken on a life of their own – and can bring their own bag of misery. Fortunately, however, fibroids often shrink and stop growing with the arrival of the menopause when oestrogen levels drop.

FRESH AND FRUITY!

Many women feel an intense rush of energy following the menopause. This can be both psychological and physical, or if you're really lucky, both! This is often called menopausal zest and marks a time when women really take stock of their lives and take a fresh look

FAREWELL TO PMS

The time has come to bid farewell to the monthly misery that is PMS! No more irritability, breast tenderness, cramps, spots or food cravings (obviously that doesn't include chocolate). Although PMS can temporarily heighten during the perimenopause as your oestrogen levels rise and fall, once that rollercoaster has come to an end it's goodbye to PMS for good!

at themselves, their own health, their relationships and the direction they next want to follow.

HEAVE HO TO HORMONAL HEADACHES!

According to the National Headache Foundation, women are affected by migraines almost three times more than men, with approximately 70 percent of these being menstrual migraines. These migraines and headaches are linked with a woman's menstruation and ovulation, and contribute greatly to the monthly misery. Fluctuating levels of progesterone and oestrogen can trigger migraines, but when these hormones fall with the arrival of the menopause, the number of hormonal headaches begins to decline.

LOOK ON THE BRIGHT SIDE

While the menopause can get some women down, it's a boost to know that, after dipping to their lowest point during the 50s, satisfaction levels rise thereafter, with women aged 69 reporting that they are the most content with their lives.

EMBRACING 'THE CHANGE'

Change is not always a bad thing, and in this case 'The Change' is a very positive time in many women's lives. Now is the perfect time to forget about any perceived flaws. You have laughter lines and things aren't as tight as they used to be, but it is confidence that is the key! Many women report a new-found self-confidence and a new opportunity to really own their sexuality as they take on the next stage in their lives. There is no way to prevent this change from happening, so embrace it and empower others to do the same.

TIME TO FOCUS ON YOURSELF

Many postmenopausal women report a great feeling of empowerment and new confidence following the biological changes in their body. After all these years of putting others first and your needs second to family and career commitments, now is the time to pursue ambitions that you might previously have been held back from. Look forward to the next adventure.

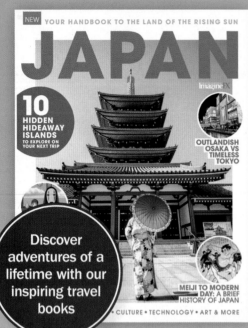

NEW — YOUR HANDBOOK TO THE LAND OF THE RISING SUN

JAPAN

ImagineFX

10 HIDDEN HIDEAWAY ISLANDS TO EXPLORE ON YOUR NEXT TRIP

OUTLANDISH OSAKA VS TIMELESS TOKYO

Discover adventures of a lifetime with our inspiring travel books

MEIJI TO MODERN DAY: A BRIEF HISTORY OF JAPAN

• CULTURE • TECHNOLOGY • ART & MORE

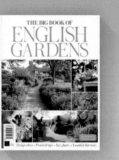

THE BIG BOOK OF
ENGLISH GARDENS

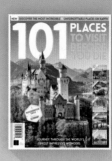

NEW — DISCOVER THE MOST INCREDIBLE — UNFORGETTABLE PLACES ON EARTH
101 PLACES TO VISIT

JOURNEY THROUGH THE WORLD'S MOST IMPRESSIVE WONDERS

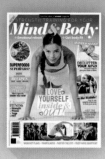

STRENGTH TRAINING FOR YOUR
Mind & Body

LOVE YOURSELF inside & OUT!

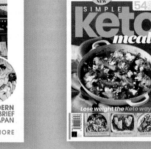

NEW — SIMPLE
keto meals

54

Lose weight the Keto way!

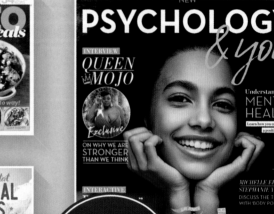
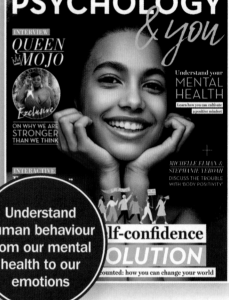

NEW
PSYCHOLOGY & you

INTERVIEW
QUEEN MOJO
Exclusive
ON WHY WE ARE STRONGER THAN WE THINK

Understand your MENTAL HEALTH
Learn how you can cultivate a positive mindset

MICHELLE ELMAN & STEPHANIE YEBOAH DISCUSS THE TROUBLE WITH 'BODY POSITIVITY'

INTERACTIVE

Self-confidence
OLUTION

Understand human behaviour from our mental health to our emotions

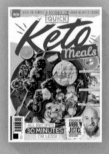

Keto meals

ALL RECIPES 30 MINUTES OR LESS!

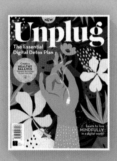

NEW
Unplug
The Essential Digital Detox Plan

Learn to live MINDFULLY in a digital world

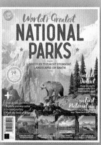

World's Greatest
NATIONAL PARKS

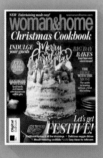

NEW — Entertaining made easy!
woman&home
Christmas Cookbook

INDULGE your guests

Let's get FESTIVE!

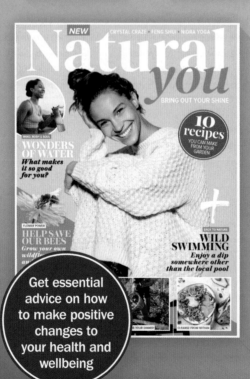

NEW — CRYSTAL CRAZE • FENG SHUI • NIDRA YOGA
Natural you
BRING OUT YOUR SHINE

10 recipes YOU CAN MAKE FROM YOUR GARDEN

WONDERS OF WATER What makes it so good for you?

HELP SAVE OUR BEES Grow your own wildlife

WILD SWIMMING Enjoy a dip somewhere other than the local pool

Get essential advice on how to make positive changes to your health and wellbeing

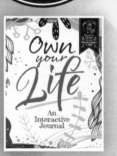

Own your Life
An Interactive Journal

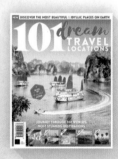

NEW — DISCOVER THE MOST BEAUTIFUL • IDYLLIC PLACES ON EARTH
101 dream TRAVEL LOCATIONS

JOURNEY THROUGH THE WORLD'S MOST STUNNING DESTINATIONS

Beginner's Guide to
Pilates

STEP-BY-STEP GUIDES for perfecting each move

Build a STRONGER you!

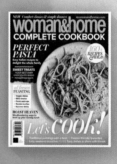

woman&home
COMPLETE COOKBOOK

PERFECT PASTA

SWEET TREATS

Let's COOK!

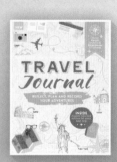

TRAVEL Journal
REFLECT, PLAN AND RECORD YOUR ADVENTURES

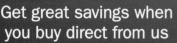

Get great savings when you buy direct from us

1000s of great titles, many not available anywhere else

World-wide delivery and super-safe ordering

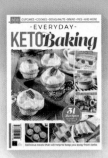
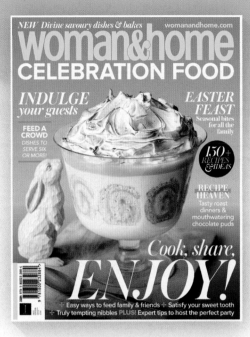
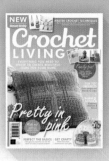
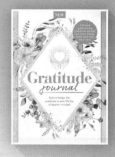
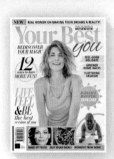
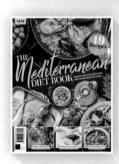
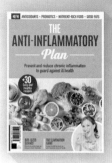
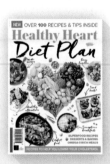
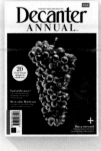
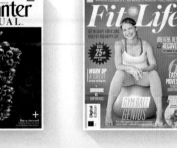
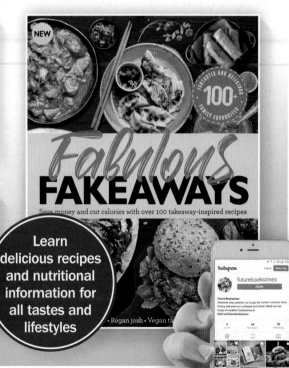
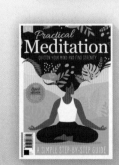
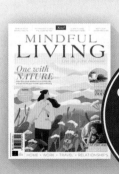
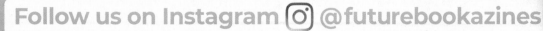
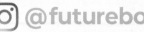

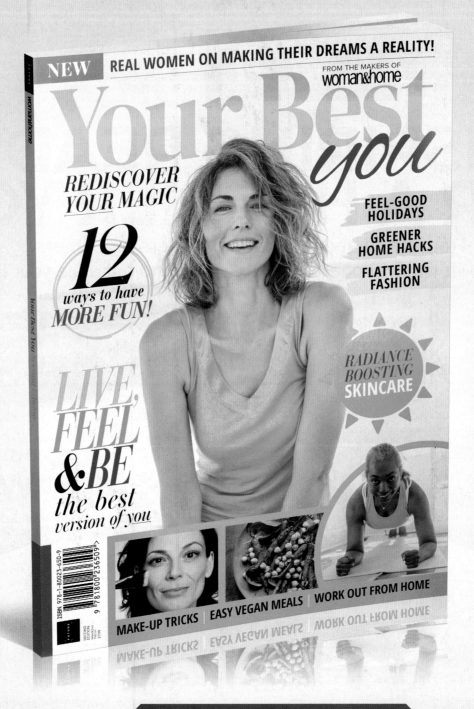